The Treatment of
Breast Cancer

The Treatment of
Breast Cancer

Edited by
Professor Sir Hedley Atkins K.B.E.

MTP
Medical and Technical Publishing Co Ltd

Published by

MTP
MEDICAL AND TECHNICAL
PUBLISHING CO LTD
PO Box 55, St Leonard's House,
St Leonardgate,
Lancaster, Lancs

ISBN-13: 978-94-011-7154-0   e-ISBN-13: 978-94-011-7152-6
DOI: 10.1007/978-94-011-7152-6

First published 1974

Produced in Great Britain by
Technical Filmsetters Europe Limited,
76 Great Bridgewater Street, Manchester M1 5JY.

Contents

List of Contributors

F. J. Ansfield, M.D., B.S.
Professor of Surgery, Cancer Research Division
University of Wisconsin, Madison, Wisconsin, U.S.A.

R. D. Bulbrook, Ph.D.
Head of the Department of Clinical Endocrinology
Imperial Cancer Research Fund,
Lincoln's Inn Fields, London WC2A 3PX

Ian Burn, F.R.C.S.
Royal Postgraduate Medical School
Hammersmith Hospital, London W12 0HS, Present Address
Charing Cross Hospital, Fulham, London W6 8RF

R. S. Handley, O.B.E., F.R.C.S.
Senior Surgeon, The Middlesex Hospital, London W1

J.-C. Heuson, M.D.
Service de Médecine et d'Investigation Clinique
Institut Jules Bordet,
Bruxelles 1000, Belgium

A. P. M. Forrest, M.D., Ch.M., F.R.C.S.
Regius Professor of Clinical Surgery
University of Edinburgh

Miss M. D. Snelling, F.R.C.P., F.R.C.S., F.F.R.
Director, Meyerstein Institute of Radiotherapy
Middlesex Hospital, London W.1

Introduction

Sir Hedley Atkins

In an article in the London *Times* of November 26th 1973 their medical correspondent, Dr Tony Smith, discussed the many methods nowadays available for the treatment of common diseases. In this article he wrote:

"Perhaps the most difficult of the common conditions is breast cancer, where the number of alternative treatments is larger than most people suppose. After the surgeon has assessed the size and nature of the growth, how far it has spread, and the general health of the woman, he has to select the optimum treatment from a range that includes simple removal of lump, removal of the breast and removal of the breast together with the underlying muscle and the lymph glands in the shoulder region. Any of these operations may be combined with various forms of X-ray treatment; or the best chance may be given by treating the tumour with high-voltage X-rays without any operation at all. Each of these treatments may give a complete cure, and, in part, the choice depends on the surgeon's skill in assessing the type of cancer present and how far it is advanced.

"The other element in the surgeon's choice, however, is his preference for one operation rather than another based on his experience and his interpretation of the results obtained by other surgical teams. Every year dozens of accounts of treatment of breast cancer are published in medical journals in Britain, the United States, and other western countries, and part of the work of a practical surgeon is reading these accounts and comparing the results with his own."

1

If "part of the work of a surgeon is reading these accounts" and, if he were to read a quarter of the literature which is poured out from the medical press each year on the subject of breast cancer, he would scarcely have time for any work. Furthermore, he would not know how to find his way through the often conflicting advice whish is showered upon him. The aim of this book is to attempt to bridge the gap between standard textbooks and research papers and to provide an assessment of the various methods available.

In dealing with a problem so complex as the treatment of breast cancer some difference of opinion is inevitably exposed in the writings of the authors of the following chapters and it would be altogether presumptuous to suppose that this book — any book — on breast cancer at this time could provide a definitive answer to the question as to what is the best method of treatment in any particular case.

Nevertheless, it might be claimed that the presently held views of great experts in their respective fields is here set out, hopefully without too many contradictory opinions, and in such a manner that a sensible answer within the range of our knowledge at this time is forthcoming. Dr Tony Smith's article refers only to early cancer, but this book deals with modern views in regard to the management of more advanced disease where treatment is directed by chemical or hormonal measures to fortify the body to resist an invasion of cancer cells far beyond the confines of the breast and the field of its lymphatic drainage.

In the first chapter, Professor Forrest literally sets the stage by describing the now frequently adopted TNM system, a more precise but slightly more complicated system than the old four stage method of categorisation familiar to senior surgeons, and one which lends itself more accurately to the prescription of treatment.

He goes on to define "cure" in this disease as the survival of the patient without evidence of disease to such a time as statistics have shown that her life expectancy is normal for her age. This conventional definition might well be set at 10 years. By such a stringent criterion the prognosis for breast cancer is not so good as many of us had supposed and he is forced to the conclusion that the method of treatment chosen for localised disease has a disappointingly small effect upon survival. This is a view which is becoming increasingly prevalent and in a later chapter, Mr R. S. Handley quotes me as saying at a meeting of the Association of Surgeons in 1953 that only in about 10% of cases does it matter what form of local treatment is chosen. If I were called upon to modify this statement in the light of a further 20 years' experience, I would not be so bold; in cancers where the axillary glands are invaded, the choice of treatment is important.

Professor Forrest discusses other problems familiar to the surgeon called upon to treat cases of breast cancer. He doubts the value of adjuvant oöphorectomy in prolonging survival in a pre-menopausal woman, as does Mr Handley; both agree that the appearance of secondaries might be delayed by this measure, but of course, at a price to her womanhood. Nevertheless, he thinks that in advanced, but still operable cases, adjuvant chemotherapy may increase the period of survival. Two common operations are contrasted, simple mastectomy (followed by immediate irradiation if the pectoral glands are found to be infiltrated, or delayed irradiation if necessary otherwise) and modified radical mastectomy as described by Patey.

Professor Forrest opts for simple mastectomy and in the next chapter Mr Handley expresses a preference for the Patey procedure. It is not necessary for the reader to wax indignant about this slight difference of opinion between two acknowledged experts and it is impossible to conceive that the two protagonists themselves would ever come to blows over such a trivial matter — the difference is in this instance insignificant.

Professor Forrest concludes by advocating the intensification of research into the effect of hormonal and cytotoxic measures designed to exorcise the cancer cell wherever it may have got to. He emphasises that such measures must be tested as to their efficacy, can only be so tested, by the controlled clinical trial.

Mr R. S. Handley discusses surgical techniques with special reference to the *quality* of life. He further tackles the formidable problem arising from the balance of advantage of a big operation which may remove all the cancer tissue on the one hand but, if it does not, may gravely impair the immune reaction of the body to the cancer cells left behind. As has been stated he prefers the Patey operation to orthodox radical mastectomy on cosmetic grounds (quality of life) and to the extended radical of Urban on immunological grounds.

Mr Handley expresses the not unreasonable view that the immune response may be made more effective by removing the bulk of the cancerous tissue and so lightening the burden on the immune mechanism, just as in days gone by the amputation of a tuberculous knee-joint helped the concomitant pulmonary lesion to heal.

If one may be permitted a personal view, I think the closure of the essential preliminary biopsy wound before a mastectomy is better done by a tight inverting skin suture (like the sero-serous layer of an intestinal anastomosis) rather than stitching a sponge over the wound. In this chapter, the work of a surgeon is quoted whose results "have never been equalled". This always makes me somewhat dubious about the comparability of the cases studied and might perhaps have been referred to as "his published results"; there cannot after all be so much difference between us. Certainly in the careful, skilled and experienced hands of Mr Handley, I would expect results which could hardly be bettered.

Miss Snelling deals with the now controversial subject of radiotherapy. Early in her chapter she gives a short account of the theory of irradiation and enumerates the different methods by which irradiation may be delivered and the place which each takes in radiotherapy. She rightly insists that the treatment of cancer of the breast in any particular case should be determined by consultation between all concerned—surgeon, radiotherapist, physician with a special knowledge of hormone therapy and chemotherapist. Having returned from a recent conference of radiotherapists in Strasbourg her interest has clearly been stimulated by the possibility of treating breast cancer by radiotherapy alone without resort to surgery. Here she is treading on controversial ground, but controversy is the lubricant of advance. It is difficult to comment on this aspect of her thesis as no controlled clinical trial to compare this treatment with more orthodox methods has, so far as my knowledge goes, been mounted. In conformity with the wise principle that orthodox therapy should be adhered to by the generality of the medical profession until some new method has been thoroughly tested and shown to be preferable, we might at this time regard the use of radiotherapy alone, in cases otherwise suitable for surgery, as an option open to a patient who expresses vigorous reluctance to the prospect of a surgical operation and an option not readily to be despised, provided the suitable apparatus and relevant experience are available.

Her chapter concludes with valuable advice in regard to the treatment of secondary deposits at special sites such as the spine, the pleura, mediastinal glands, the brain and the eye.

Hormone therapy is discussed in two chapters. In the first, Dr Heuson deals with hormone therapy by administration, and in the second, Mr Ian Burn describes the methods available to modify the hormonal environment by ablating the ovary, the adrenal glands and the hypophysis. In the former chapter Dr Heuson compares the effects of oestrogens, androgens, progestogens and the corticosteroids together with some less commonly used hormones, and describes the indications for their use together with the side effects which each produces.

Mr Burn, like other contributors, is on the whole against routine adjuvant oöphorectomy for early cancers treated by surgery, although he admits that this operation might delay the appearance of recurrences without affecting survival. In the advanced case in a pre-menopausal woman he prefers surgical obliteration of the hormonal influence of the ovaries rather than achieving this by irradiation, if only because the former method allows examination of the liver at laparotomy.

He discusses the hoary problem of the relative advantages of adrenalectomy and hypophysectomy, two operations where the indications are virtually the same, but reserves judgement, and well he might. The results of recent controlled clinical trials seem to lend credence to the view that, where the necessary and highly individual expertise is available, hypophysectomy holds a slight but significant advantage over adrenalectomy. Where this is not available, to opt for hypophysectomy is disastrous.

In a short chapter on chemotherapy Dr Ansfield recommends 5-Fluorouracil as the sheet-anchor of the cytotoxic approach. He is quite unequivocal on this matter, no doubt to the relief of the reader, and gives cogent reasons for his choice. He is resolutely opposed to the use of alkylating drugs first because they render subsequent hormone therapy ineffective, and second because of the severe effect which these drugs have on the bone marrow. Because 5-Fluorouracil does not have the former effect he is able to recommend its use before adrenalectomy or hypophysectomy in the advanced case. A possible disadvantage to this sequence is that, while waiting to see whether the drug will work, the patient's condition might deteriorate to the extent that one or other of these major operations becomes impracticable. If the operation is done first, the drug can always be administered later.

In reading accounts of the treatment of breast cancer from the United States, it must be remembered that almost all their cases have had a radical mastectomy, thus, when Dr Ansfield recommends the use of adjuvant cytotoxic therapy if "more than four axillary nodes" are found to be invaded after operation, this recommendation must be modified in Forrest's cases so that this adjuvant therapy is advocated where a pectoral gland only is found to be invaded.

Dr Ansfield never gives up, and considerable clinical and humane judgement is required in the moribund case to decide whether a kindly prescription of opiates is to be preferred to a cytotoxic cocktail during the last days. Such a decision might have to depend upon testamentory considerations, and it must be remembered that heroin has not been available therapeutically in the United States for many years.

In the final chapter, Dr R. D. Bulbrook covers the vital issue of predictive factors. To have information about how a patient is likely to behave is important enough in itself but a study of those factors which may betoken a favourable response to remedial measures may lead to fundamental knowledge about the causes of the cancer, and so to the elaboration of more specific and thus more effective treatment so that the first three chapters of this book dealing with local treatments become of historic interest only.

Dr Bulbrook deals with the predictive values of stage and grade, characteristics which have been recognised as of prognostic importance for many decades. He refers to the more recently appreciated indicators such as the menopausal status and the free period, the latter a measure of the interval between the original treatment and the first appearance of secondaries and so of the rate of development of the cancer.

The predictive factors discussed, concurrently serve two functions. The first indicates the natural history which any particular case is likely to pursue; the second, the probable response to treatment, these two functions being in most cases positively correlated. The second function—response to treatment—has been applied particularly to the more recently discovered predictive factors such as the pattern of steroid excretion in the urine.

He concludes by describing more sophisticated predictors which are now being extensively investigated such as receptor sites, tryptophan metabolism, the ability of tumour tissue to sulphate steroids and the carcino-embryonic antigen.

Advances in this field are so rapid and the necessity for expansion of our knowledge so urgent that we must expect and hope that some of the latter part of this chapter will, within the course of the next few years, have to be rewritten, a consequence devoutly to be consummated so that cancer of the breast joins with tuberculosis, typhoid and tetanus as a disease over which mankind has provided himself with the tools of mastery.

1

Primary cancer of the breast — indications for therapy

A. P. M. Forrest

The objective in treating cancer of the breast is cure. In practice this implies control of local disease and prevention of dissemination.

In this chapter we will first look at current orthodox practice and examine its success at achieving this objective; we will consider which factors may influence this and then discuss the changes in therapy which must take place if we are ever to improve the appalling results.

Orthodox treatment of primary breast cancer and its assessment

The management of a patient with a primary cancer of the breast is in 3 parts: diagnosis, assessment of extent, and treatment. For the first, clinical examination followed by excision biopsy at the time of mastectomy are still orthodox practice. The assessment of operability is also still based on clinical and radiological findings and leads to the clinical staging of the disease. That most frequently used is the UICC international system based on characteristics of tumour (T), its related lymph nodes (N), and the presence or absence of systemic metastatic spread (M). These can be conveniently assessed by the use of a precoded form. That shown in Figure 1.1 and the following notes are based on the 1960 classification.

Tumour

The T category of a tumour is determined by size, extent of invasion of surrounding tissue and lymphoedema. If less than 2.5 cm in diameter it is classified T1, if 2.5–5.0 cm T2, if 5–10 cm T3, and over 10 cm T4. Fixation to overlying skin, if incomplete, is T2, if complete, but within the confines of the tumour T3, if wide of this T4. Fixation to underlying pectoral muscle is

9

TNM STAGING

PRIMARY TUMOUR

Size	Skin fixation	Peau d'orange	Paget's disease	Nipple retraction	Pectoral muscle fixation	Chest wall fixation	Category	Stage
Not more than 2cm ☐	None ☐	None ☐	None / Nipple only	None ☐	None ☐	None ☐	T₁	1
More than 2cm not more than 5cm ☐	Incomplete (tethered or dimpled) ☐		Extending beyond nipple	Present ☐			T₂	
More than 5cm not more than 10cm ☐	Complete (infiltrated or ulcerated) ☐	In tumour area only ☐			Present ☐		T₃	3
More than 10cm ☐	Wide of tumour but not beyond breast area ☐	Wide of tumour but within breast ☐				Present ☐	T₄	

RADIOLOGY   date   no mets   mets

Chest (lungs)   Chest (ribs)   Skull   Pelvis   Spine   Mammogram   Scintigram

REGIONAL LYMPH NODES

Ipsilateral axillary nodes	Supra & Infra clavicular nodes	Oedema of arm	Category	Stage
Not palpable ☐	Not palpable ☐	None ☐	N₀	1
Palpable but mobile ☐ Single ☐ Multiple ☐	Considered to contain growth [yes	no]		N₁A	1
			N₁B	2
Fixed to one another ☐ Fixed to other structures ☐			N₂	3
	Moveable ☐ Fixed ☐	Present ☐	N₃	

BIOPSY

Primary tumour   date   pos   neg

Needle   Drill   Open

DISTANT METASTASES

		Category	Stage
Skin involvement wide of the breast ☐	None ☐	M₀	1
the contralateral lymph nodes or breast ☐	Present ☐	M₁	4
clinical or radiological evidence of metastases to lungs, pleural cavity, skeleton, liver, brain, etc ☐	Name of Dr completing form and date of examination		

Figure 1.1   TNM Staging Form. (Note: Scintigrum is not used for clinical staging)

T3, to chest wall T4. Lymphoedema within the confines of a tumour makes it T3, if wide of it T4.

Nodes

Regional nodes are graded N0 to N3 according to palpability, fixation and extent of involvement. If no nodes are palpable, it is N0, if mobile nodes are felt in the homolateral axilla N1, if these are fixed N2. If nodes are palpated in the contralateral axilla or in the supraclavicular region, or if enlargement of ipsilateral nodes is associated with arm oedema, the grade is N3.

Metastases

This is M0 or M1 according to whether distant metastases are absent or present. In the asymptomatic patient, the investigation for these routinely includes X-rays of the chest and selected bones. We normally restrict these to ribs, skull and pelvis, but also include mammography of the other breast.

STAGING

As a result of these criteria, patients are classified into one of four international stages. Early disease limited to the breast (T1 or T2, N0, M0) is stage 1; if accompanied by palpable but mobile axillary nodes (T1 or T2, N1, M0) Stage 2. Stage 3 is locally advanced disease (T3 or T4, N2 or N3, M0); and Stage 4 the presence of distant metastases.

Orthodox therapy is based on clinical staging as follows.

Stages 1 and 2

These patients are accepted as having "curable" breast cancer; the aim of primary treatment is to eradicate the disease. A whole range of surgical procedures has been used for this purpose. At one end of the spectrum is local excision of the tumour; at the other, super-radical operations in which the pectoral muscles, axillary, supraclavicular and internal mammary lymph nodes are removed en bloc. Between are simple or total mastectomy; a series of "modified radical" operations, in which the breast and varying proportions of the axillary contents are removed in continuity; the "classical radical" mastectomy in which the pectoral muscles also are removed; and extended radical mastectomy, which includes also resection of the internal mammary chain. Radiotherapy may be used to supplement surgical treatment, particularly when this has been of less radical type, but only rarely is the sole method of treatment for "operable" disease.

Two recent surveys indicate the extent to which practice varies in Britain and in the United States (Table 1.1). In general this consists of either a radical resection of the breast and axillary nodes in continuity, or removal of the breast alone with post-operative radical radiotherapy to local lymph nodes. Additional therapy, either endocrine or chemotherapeutic, is not commonly used and is virtually limited to those whose axillary lymph nodes are believed to be involved. British surgeons tend to be more conservative when the tumour is on the medial side of the breast, local mastectomy and radiotherapy being the preferred procedure in the majority of cases.

Stage 3

Orthodox primary treatment for stage 3 (locally advanced) cancer of the breast aims to control local disease. Although it is not generally accepted that cure is possible, some of these

Table 1.1 RESULTS OF SURVEYS REPORTED BY FORREST[1] AND NEMOTO[2] USING THE SAME QUESTIONNAIRE TO DETERMINE THE METHODS USED TO TREAT CANCER OF THE BREAST OF 3 HYPOTHETICAL TYPES

	%	
	UK	NY
Surgery		
superradical	< 1	1
classical radical	21	77
modified radical	33	17
simple	41	5
local excision	5	—
none	< 1	—
Radiotherapy		
advised	31	26
decision left to		
radiotherapist	36	22
not advised	33	52
Adjuvant therapy		
ovariectomy	24	27
chemotherapy	4	2
none	67	67

Opinions of 415 British and 92 North American surgeons on treatment of primary cancer of the breast (Stages 1 and 2) in premenopausal patients

patients belong to a favourable group when the tumours have become locally advanced only because of their low metastasising potential. Control of local disease may be associated with survival for long periods of time. In most instances "radical" radiotherapy is best.

On occasions, toilet surgery by wide excision or by a local mastectomy, may usefully precede radiotherapy or be used for residual disease after primary treatment. This is indicated only if tumour tissue is not transgressed, e.g. those tumours classified T3 on the basis of size alone.

The place of systemic therapy for T3 tumours has never properly been assessed. Yet elderly patients may have longstanding regression of disease from the administration of hormones alone.

Stage 4
Palliation of symptoms is the general aim of therapy. When

distant metastases are present, local treatment is contra-indicated except for the local control of ulcerating or fungating lesions; then radiotherapy is preferred. As adequate systemic treatment will also control the primary tumour, there is no indication to use local therapy until this has been assessed. Further consideration of Stage 3 and 4 cases will be found in Chapter 00. Here we are concerned with "curable" tumours, those currently designated as Stages 1 and 2.

Success in achieving objectives
The measure of success of orthodox therapy in patients with Stage 1 and 2 cancer is the proportion cured of their disease. Most surgeons accept that the absence of local recurrence or of dissemination during the remainder of a patient's life-time is indicative of cure; strictly it should also include absence of disease at death. This stringent criterion can rarely be applied. Patients treated for breast cancer, and who apparently die from other causes, rarely have post mortems. Yet without autopsy evidence, certified causes of death can be inaccurate. Death from metastases in the myocardium or lungs may be recorded "cardiac failure"; from metastases in bone marrow, "chronic anaemia", or in liver "general debility".

SURVIVAL
Cure is also assessed by survival statistics at defined times after treatment. Five-year survival rates are of no value in assessing cure of a disease when first evidence of recurrence may be 20–30 years later. A more useful guide is the time when the annual death rate of patients with the disease no longer exceeds significantly that of the normal population[3,92]. In breast cancer this occurs around 15 years after treatment. Although patients may still die from recurrence after this time, 15-year survival rates give a reasonable guide to what is achieved.

Such rates for all cases of primary operable cancer of the breast treated within a defined geographical area are seldom available. The results of several large series of selected cases suggest that it does not exceed 30%. This figure represents the results of treating early and curable cases; not that of all cases of breast cancer. According to the study reported by Brinkley and

Haybittle[92], crude 15-year survival of all cases was 17%, and age-corrected 24%.

In general terms, 4 out of 5 patients seen with cancer of the breast will die from their disease within fifteen years; of those initially considered curable, at least $\frac{2}{3}$ will share the same fate. These depressing results are due to the simple fact that local therapy can prevent dissemination of the disease only if it precedes extension beyond the primary site. It can never cure disease which is already generalised.

RESULTS OF UNTREATED CASES

It is appropriate to consider the proportion of patients who survive for the same length of time without treatment. The most complete study was that of Bloom[4], who reviewed the fate of 1728 patients reported from various centres with untreated breast cancer. Fifteen-year survival rates were available for 476 patients; only 3 lived. The 10-year survival rate for 657 cases was 5%.

This study included Bloom's own series of 250 cases observed at the Middlesex Charity between 1805 and 1933, from which histological material was available. Although 97% were advanced when first seen, the similar distribution of the nuclear grade to that found in more recent series of treated cases suggested that no particular factor of selection was involved.

LOCAL RECURRENCE

A second method to assess success of primary treatment is by control of local disease. The pattern of local recurrence varies from the small nodule of recurrent tumour in the line of the scar, due to continued growth of odd clusters of cells; to extensive diffuse infiltration encompassing the chest in a "cuirasse" or causing widespread superficial ulceration and due to invasion of dermal lymphatics or capillaries. This distinction is seldom made when local recurrence rates are defined; in fact most also include recurrence in regional lymph nodes.

Local recurrence is due to residual cancer in skin flaps. According to Auchincloss[5] cancer cells in the dermis can be recognised in 9% of radical mastectomy specimens.

The incidence of local recurrence after orthodox therapy varies. In a study of 507 patients in whom radical mastectomy had failed to cure the disease, Collins[6] reported that $\frac{1}{4}$ had first evidence of recurrence locally. A local recurrence rate of 30% over 10 years was reported in a series of 433 cases treated in Edinburgh by simple mastectomy and radiotherapy[7,8]. In these cases again, local recurrence usually heralded the development of disseminated disease. In the Manchester trial (see below), the local recurrence rate in those treated by radical mastectomy alone, was 32%. However, the proportion of patients in whom local recurrence was uncontrolled at death, was 15%.

It can be concluded that in the majority of patients with breast cancer of Stage 1 and 2, orthodox local therapy can control local disease. However, those patients who develop local recurrence usually die from disseminated disease, a fact indicating the need for its treatment by systemic as well as local therapy.

TYPE OF LOCAL TREATMENT
It is pertinent to consider whether the type of local therapy materially affects these results. Retrospective comparisons help little. Unless one includes all cases of disease arising in a defined population, one cannot account for the effect of selection of cases. As was shown in a comparison of patients treated in private and public sectors of the hospital service, this can be profound[9].

The results of prospective controlled randomised trials are more valid and are considered under several heads.

Radical mastectomy versus simple mastectomy and radiotherapy
Three trials have compared radical surgery with simple mastectomy and radiotherapy using the McWhirter regime of 4500 rad over 3 weeks. Recurrence-free survival rates have been identical.

In that from Copenhagen, which included 666 patients, the radical mastectomy was of extended type, including removal of the breast, pectoral muscles, axillary, supraclavicular and internal mammary lymph nodes. Ten-year survival rates were the same as in patients treated by the simple regime[10]. This trial has been criticised on the grounds that both groups of patients included a proportion of inoperable cases, as well as some patients who were not treated strictly according to protocol. However the results were not influenced by their exclusion.

The Cambridge trial was limited to patients with palpable axillary nodes. The radical mastectomy was of Halsted type and this also was followed by radical radiotherapy. In the simple mastectomy group, surgeons were allowed to remove accessible nodes but did not formally dissect the axilla. Six-year results were reported in 113 patients[11]. There were no significant differences, but a slight trend in favour of the simpler procedure.

The Edinburgh trial started in 1964 and also used a classical radical mastectomy without post-operative radiotherapy, which was compared with the standard Edinburgh regime of simple mastectomy and radiotherapy. The preliminary 5-year results in 203 patients have revealed no differences[12].

Extension of local therapy beyond the breast and axilla
Although the results of super-radical surgery, in the hands of Urban, are impressive, several controlled randomised studies indicate that extension of local treatment beyond the breast and axilla whether by surgery or radiotherapy does not improve survival rates. One of these from Copenhagen, which compared extension of standard surgical radical mastectomy by surgical removal of internal mammary and supraclavicular nodes, has already been discussed above.

Two trials have examined the effects of adding radiotherapy to the standard radical operation, the object being to control residual local disease.

That from Manchester was the first controlled trial to be carried out in patients with breast cancer[13]. It included 1461 patients treated by radical mastectomy between 1948 and 1952, and was aimed at determining if routine post-operative radiotherapy conferred any advantage over a watching policy in which radiotherapy was used when local recurrence developed. Two techniques of radiotherapy were studied: to the anterior chest wall and axilla alone (720 patients) and to the axilla, supraclavicular fossa and internal mammary chain (741 patients).

Ten-year survival rates were identical both for the total groups (which included a small proportion of Stage 3 cancers) and those with histologically proved Stages 1 and 2 cancer. Although the incidence of local recurrence was reduced by post-operative radiotherapy, this was equally well controlled in the watched group if therapy was given when local recurrence developed. The number of patients in the treated and watched groups who had local recurrence at death was identical[14].

A similar conclusion was reached in a study conducted by the National Surgical Adjuvant Breast Project (NSABP) team in the United States. 1103 patients treated by radical mastectomy were included; 470 received parasternal, axillary and supraclavicular irradiation, 633 were controls. Despite the significant reduction in regional and local recurrence rates, the fate of the patients at 5 years was identical, irrespective of axillary node status at the time of primary treatment[15].

Conservative local therapy
Two trials are under way in Britain to assess whether simple mastectomy alone is justifiable treatment for primary breast cancer. These are considered in the third section of this chapter.

A trial in which local excision of the tumour was the surgical procedure under test was reported from Guy's Hospital[16]. 370 patients with breast cancer of Stages 1 and 2 were included; 188 were treated by classical radical mastectomy; 182 by postoperative radiotherapy, but the form of this varied. In the radical group, 3000 rad were given to regional lymph node fields by conventional (250 kV) apparatus; in the local excision group, 3800 rad were given to the breast and internal mammary chain by linear accelerator, and 3000 rad to axillary and supraclavicular areas by orthodox therapy. Both groups of patients included early in the trial were also given a short course of thio-TEPA of total dose 0.7 mg per kg body weight over 4 days.

In those with clinically palpable axillary nodes, the incidence of local and distant recurrence in those patients treated by local excision proved to be significantly higher and 5- and 10-year survival rates significantly lower than in those treated by radical mastectomy. In patients without palpable nodes, local excision, although still followed by a higher incidence of local and axillary recurrence, resulted in better survival rates.

Although Atkins and his colleagues suggest that clinically involved axillary nodes are best removed at the time of primary operation, the trial has been criticised on the grounds that the dose of radiotherapy given to the axilla in the local excision group would nowadays be regarded as insufficient.

Radical or modified radical mastectomy

The standard radical mastectomy of Halsted involves sacrifice of the pectoralis major muscle. Its functions are dichotomous in that its clavicular part which usually is preserved in a radical mastectomy, acts with the anterior portion of the deltoid to raise the arm forward and to control its descent. The larger costal part, which normally is removed, acts in concert with latissimus dorsi and teres major to pull the arm down against resistance, or if the arm is fixed as in climbing, to raise the trunk. For the average woman removal of this muscle causes little functional disability. In the study of 507 patients by Watson *et al.*[17], severe loss of function was experienced by only 1.9%.

Of greater consequence is the loss of the muscle pad, particularly below the clavicle, which can lead to an unsightly hollow; and the loss of muscle supporting the wearing of an ordinary brassière.

Most British surgeons now follow the lead of Patey and his colleagues from the Middlesex Hospital, and preserve this muscle. There are no randomised controlled trials by which one can assess the safety of this procedure. However, one can examine the validity of the reasons given in preference for the Halsted operation. These are the eradication of lymphatic pathways and the facilitation of access to the axilla.

(i) Lymphatic pathways. The classical belief that an important lymphatic plexus runs in close relationship to the fascia covering the pectoral muscle has not been supported by recent studies, in which *in vivo* injections of dyes and radioisotopes have been used to map out the lymphatic drainage of the breast[18,19]. The main lymphatics draining the breast run within its substance towards the axilla and perforate the deep fascia with the axillary tail. The few fine channels which run deep to the breast in the pectoral fascia probably only drain the fascia itself. Lymphatics from the breast do perforate the deep fascia other than in the axilla, but only at certain focal points and then by accompanying the perforating branches of the internal mammary and inter-costal vessels. Such lymphatics gain entry to the thoracic cavity and drain into intrathoracic nodes. The only exception is in the upper part of the chest, where some lymphatics pass through the pectoral muscles with the acromio-thoracic vessels to drain into the inter-pectoral nodes of Rotter. Apart from removal of these small and probably insignificant nodes, excision of the pectoral muscle mass does not give added protection.

(ii) Access to axilla. There are now several studies indicating that removal of the pectoralis major muscle is not an essential step to gain full access to the axilla. As was reported by Patey and Dyson[20], lifting the arm so that the forearm lies in front of and parallel to the chest, and the upper arm at right angles to it, relaxes the pectoralis major muscle which can be retracted to expose the pectoralis minor. When this is divided the upper reaches of the axilla are in full view. Lymphangiographic studies have indicated that the axilla can thus be completely cleared of lymph nodes[21].

In any case the relationship of axillary node involvement to the prognosis of breast cancer suggests that high axillary clearance is a fruitless surgical exercise.

ADDITIONAL THERAPY

Realisation of the frequency with which primary operable breast cancer is already generalised has led to an examination of the value of additional systemic therapy, this having as its object the destruction of residual systemic disease. The methods used include endocrine therapy and chemotherapy.

Endocrine therapy

(i) Prophylactic castration. Two trials to assess the value of prophylactic castration at the time of orthodox primary treat-ment have been reported. That from Manchester included 596 pre-menopausal women, who following radical mastectomy were allocated randomly for irradiation of each ovary with 450 rad, or to a control group in which no additional therapy was given[22]. That from Oslo included a total of 910 pre-menopausal and post-menopausal women. Randomised com-parisons were carried out between surgical castration and ovarian irradiation (1000 rad to each ovary) in pre-menopausal

women with Stage 2 cancer; and between local treatment alone
and local treatment supplemented by ovarian irradiation in
pre-menopausal women with Stage 1 cancer, and ˙post-
menopausal women with Stages 1 and 2 cancer[23]. Both trials
indicated that prophylactic oöphorectomy or ovarian irradiation postpones the onset of recurrent disease. According to
Nissen-Meyer, it also leads to an absolute prolongation of survival in both pre- and post-menopausal women. This view is
not supported by Cole, who found that the prompt use of
therapeutic castration at the time of recurrence˙ had no
effect on survival rates.

According to Fisher[15], the 3-year results of the NSABP
trial of prophylactic castration in 357 women do not give any
justification for its use in operable cancer of the breast.

This view is accepted by most British surgeons, who advocate prophylactic castration only when the disease is manifestly
incurable. As it can benefit only those with hormone sensitive
tumours; even then it is bound to fail to benefit the majority of
women.

(ii) Other endocrine measures. In 1960, Patey[24] treated a small
series of post-menopausal patients whose axillary nodes contained tumour by adding prophylactic adrenalectomy to their
primary treatment. He did not find any advantage. More
recently Dao et al.[25], have advocated a similar policy of treatment in those with 4 or more nodes involved.

Additive endocrine therapy by the implant of 200 mg
testosterone at the time of mastectomy and subsequently at 9-
month intervals is under trial in Toronto. No significant results
have yet been published[26]. The principle underlying this treatment was the poor prognosis in those women who, at the time
of mastectomy, excreted abnormally low amounts of aetiocholanolone in the urine.

For many years therapy with thyroid extract was believed
to be of value to patients with breast cancer. A controlled randomised study of prophylactic thyroid therapy in 217 patients
with mammary cancer treated by simple mastectomy and
radiotherapy proved it to be of no value in the dose used[27].

Chemotherapy
Several controlled randomised studies of the value of prophy-

lactic chemotherapy have been reported from the United States[15]. In these the chemotherapeutic agent was given only for a short period post-operatively. An advantage was conferred only in pre-menopausal patients with positive axillary nodes, possibly due to the effect of the drug on the ovaries. Postmenopausal patients did not derive benefit.

Longer term chemotherapy is also under study. A small controlled trial was recently reported by Riache et al.[28], in which cyclophosphamide 200 mg per day was started at the time of surgery and continued until a total dose of 100 mg per kg body weight had been given. In those patients with positive axillary nodes at the time of operation, 3-year survival and local recurrence rates were significantly better than in control patients. Similar results have been reported by Nissen–Meyer et al.[30]. This form of additional therapy will further be considered below.

CONCLUSION
It is clear that orthodox local therapy fails to control the disease in the majority of patients treated; most patients who die from the disease do so with metastases present. Local therapy can prevent dissemination only if it precedes extension of the disease beyond the primary site. It can never cure disease which is already generalised. Arguments as to the best form of local therapy cannot make any impact on the curability of breast cancer and energy should rather be expended on a reappraisal of our whole policy of management.

Other prognostic factors
It is not only the type of treatment which influences the curability of cancer of the breast. Other factors are concerned and will be considered in this section under biology, extent of disease and the influence of delay in treatment.

BIOLOGY
Background of patient
Several excellent reviews of demographic and endocrine influences on the risk of a woman developing cancer of the breast have recently been published[30-32]. Of these the most important is age at first pregnancy: the risk of breast cancer in women in South Wales whose first child was born before the age of 18

years was half that of those who first became pregnant when
40 or more[33]. The influence of these factors on the prognosis of
established disease is less well defined.
(i) Age. In contrast to general belief, cancer of the breast does
not carry an unduly bad prognosis in the young. Pre-menopausal women have survival rates equal if not better than those
in women past the menopause. The natural cessation of ovarian
function which occurs at the time of the menopause may contribute by inducing a period of tumour inactivity. Several
studies have shown that when the menopause intervenes between primary treatment and first recurrence of disease the
duration of the free interval is longer than when both occur
either in the pre- or post-menopausal period.
(ii) Castration. Women whose ovaries have been removed in
youth have a lower incidence of breast cancer than those whose
reproductive organs are intact[31]. Also castrated women who
develop the disease have a more favourable prognosis[34]. As
indicated above, oöphorectomy or ovarian irradiation, performed at the time of primary treatment, delays the onset of
recurrent disease.
(iii) Pregnancy. The prognosis of cancer of the breast occurring
during pregnancy is not as severe as was once believed. In a
recent study of 220 women whose breast cancer appeared concurrently with pregnancy, Peters[35] found no evidence to support the accepted view that pregnancy had a deleterious effect
on the natural history of the disease, other than in those women
whose cancers were discovered and treated during its second
half. Nor does a pregnancy subsequent to the treatment of
cancer of the breast worsen survival rates. In fact the converse
may be true. The survival rates of 96 women who became pregnant after the treatment of breast cancer were reported by
Peters to be 28% better at 10 years than those in controls
matched for age and stage of disease. This improvement was
most pronounced in women under 35 years of age.
    Although it has been suggested that only those women
with favourable disease will survive to become pregnant, this is
not likely to be the sole reason for the difference observed by
Peters, 50% of the pregnancies in her series occurred within 1,
and 75% within 2 years of initial treatment.
(iv) Urinary steroids. According to Bulbrook and his associates

at the Imperial Cancer Research Laboratories, patients with breast cancer, who at the time of mastectomy excrete abnormally low amounts of the C-19 steroid metabolite aetiocholanolone in the urine, have a worse prognosis than those with normal outputs of this steroid. In their studies the proportion of urinary aetiocholanolone to that of 17-hydroxycorticosteroids, metabolites of the C-21 steroids (glucocorticoids) was expressed as a "discriminant function", initially designed as an index of prediction of response of patients with advanced breast cancer to hypophysectomy or adrenalectomy. The 8-year cumulative survival curves for those patients with negative discriminants (low aetiocholanolone excretion) were reported by Hayward et al.[36] to be less favourable than in those in whom this was positive (normal aetiocholanolone excretion). This finding has not been confirmed.

THE TUMOUR

Certain features of a mammary tumour influence its prognosis. With the exception of a medullary cancer the basic morphology of an infiltrative tumour is relatively unimportant, but the degree of anaplasia, the contour of the tumour, and lymphocytic infiltration do influence survival rates.

Tumour grade

The histological grade of a tumour can be assessed by the degree of tubular differentiation, the regularity of size and shape of the nuclei and their staining properties, and the frequency of mitotic figures[37]. Three grades of tumour have been defined and these have been related to prognosis. In tumours of Grade 1, i.e. the most differentiated, survival rates are 2–3 times greater than in those of Grade 3[38]. Most of the deaths in patients with Grade 3 tumours occur within the first 5 years.

An alternative system of grading used by Cutler and his associates[39] is based on nuclear characteristics only. At one end of the spectrum the nuclei are similar in size and appearance both to one another and also to those found in normal duct cells; at the other they are irregular and enlarged with prominent nucleoli and clumping of chromatin. These changes also have been related to survival.

The relationship between the histological grade of a tumour and its prognosis is not as simple as may first appear.

For example, the medullary cancer on account of its florid anaplasia is included in Bloom's Grade 3; yet this tumour has a
prognosis similar to those of Grade 1[40]. There is also the difficulty of precise allocation of tumours within an arbitrary 3-
point scale. The relationship between grade and prognosis can
be materially altered by the direction in which indeterminate
tumours on the border zones are put[41]. The main value of
grading has been in retrospective studies when it can be used to
.assess comparability of tumours. As the variation of grade in
different parts of the same tumour makes representative grading
of small samples out of the question, it is unlikely to prove of
value in determining prospectively the form of surgical treatment.

Contour
Primary cancers of the breast can be grouped according to their
contour determined by mammography or by histological
preparations of whole slices of removed breasts. Using both
techniques, we defined 4 types of contour: (i) smooth or circumscribed; (ii) irregular or spiculated; (iii) mixed, in which both
smooth and spiculated areas were present and; (iv) con-
glomerate, a mulberry-like contour[42]. The relationship between contour and prognosis was first described by Ingleby and
Gershon–Cohen[43]. In a mammographic study of 295 tumours,
they found that the .3-year survival rates for those with circumscribed tumours (63%) were better than for those whose
tumours had an irregular contour (41%). Similar findings were
described by Lane and his colleagues[44], who assessed contour
on the naked-eye appearance of cut mastectomy specimens.
Ten-year survival rates for 44 patients with tumours with circumscribed outlines were 80%; for 158 patients with irregular
tumours, 38%.

By contrast we found no significant relationship between
contour type and clinical or mammographic stage of the disease,
the size of the tumour, its histological grade, or the presence of
axillary node involvement[42].

Elastosis
The semi-quantitative assessment of the degree of elastosis in a
series of 103 patients was found to provide a reliable guide to the

prognosis of primary breast cancer[45]. This elastic tissue, when present invests groups of tumour cells and when dense constitute a salient histological feature in some tumours. Ultrastructural studies have indicated that the elastica is produced by the neoplastic epithelial cells.

Round cell infiltration

In 1955, Black and Speer[46] described the good prognosis associated with infiltration of a breast cancer with round cells. This reaction occurs within the interstices of cords of tumour, particularly at its advancing edge. Axillary node involvement is less common and survival rates are better when this change is marked[39,47,48]. Frequently reported in tumours with primitive nuclear grades, it is most pronounced in medullary cancers.

Many regard round cell infiltration of immunological significance. This is supported by the findings that those patients with infiltrated tumours of several types more frequently show a delayed hypersensitivity response to the intradermal injection of isologous and homologous breast tumour extracts than those without[49].

Round cell infiltrates include both lymphocytes and plasma cells. These are now considered to represent separate parts of the immune system. The former, T-cells, are concerned with cell-mediated immunity; the latter, B-cells, with the production of circulating antibodies. Estimations of immunoglobulins in tumour eluates indicate that those from tumours with a marked plasma cell infiltrate contain higher concentrations of IgM than those with no such infiltrate[50].

Medullary cancer

This is a rare tumour accounting for under 3% of all breast cancers. Its most striking clinical feature is its circumscribed outline and even when large its apparent encapsulation. It is soft, bulky and frequently associated with redness and oedema of the overlying skin, features which give it a highly malignant appearance. Microscopically, it also looks strikingly malignant. A degenerate stroma surrounds strands and masses of large and sometimes bizarre cell forms which are highly anaplastic. Characteristic is the zone of circulating fibrosis and the prominent lymphocytic infiltration. Despite their sinister appearance, medullary cancers have a particularly good prognosis and Bloom[52], suggests that the best treatment is radical surgery.

Two features of the medullary cancer, its circumscribed outline and its lymphocytic infiltration, have been already described to influence favourably the prognosis of breast cancer. It is tempting to believe that it is those factors which give a medullary tumour an outlook which considering its anaplasia is unique.

IMMUNE RESPONSES

Reaction in regional lymph nodes

Palpable enlargement of homolateral axillary lymph nodes not involved by metastatic disease and of those in the contralateral axilla is associated with improved survival rates from breast cancer, particularly in large tumours[39,53]. A specific histological change, termed sinus histiocytosis, has been described in the regional lymph nodes of patients with cancer, and is believed to be reactive in nature. The sinusoids of the lymph nodes are dilated and distended with large elongated cells with distinctive eosinophilic cytoplasm. Elsewhere the node contains closely packed lymphoid cells which blur the normal difference between cortex and medulla. Several reports have confirmed the original observation of Black and his colleagues[54] that this change also favourably affects prognosis. In patients in which it is marked, survival rates are uncommonly good. For example, in a study of 217 patients with primary breast cancer followed for 10 years, Daoud[55] found a survival rate of 85% in those which marked sinus histiocytosis compared to 12% when this change was not present. Recently Good[56] has reported that the converse is also true; depletion of lymphocytes in regional lymph nodes is a bad prognostic sign.

Immunological response

Until a decade ago, there was only sparse information about the ability of a patient to react immunologically to a breast cancer. Such tests of cellular immune function as were used were non-specific: for example, the delayed hypersensitivity response to tuberculin or streptokinase or *in vitro* transformation of lymphocytes following their exposure to the mitogen phytohaemagglutinin. Such studies mainly serve to show that loss of ability to react to a non-specific stimulus decreased as the disease progressed. The persistence of normal lymphocyte transformation *in vitro* suggested that progression of cancer might be associated with a growing lack of recognition of an antigenic stimulus.

Recently attention has been turned to more specific tests of immune function. These include challenge of a patient with her own tumour, the detection of sensitisation of lymphocytes to it, or the presence of circulating antibodies which react against it. These have provided evidence that immune recognition of a tumour does occur, at least in a proportion of patients.

That initially reported by Hughes and MacKay[57] was of delayed hypersensitivity reactions by patients to their own tumor when this was injected intradermally. Since then more sophisticated *in vitro* tests of cell-bound immunity, e.g. macrophage inhibition, lymphocyte transformation and cytotoxicity have tended to confirm this. From work in this department, Roberts[93], has reported that patients with primary breast cancer may show evidence of depression of recognition of a foreign antigen and that approximately $\frac{1}{2}$ of them will show evidence of cell-bound immunity to their own tumour. This has also been demonstrated in a small percentage of patients with fibroadenomas.

These tests are of T-cell function and do not take into account the activity of the B-cells which are responsible for the production of circulating antibodies. There is little work worthy of note in this field. In a recent study by Roberts[94], evidence for precipitating antibodies to tumour was demonstrated in 10% of patients with operable cancer of the breast.

The relationship of these responses to prognosis is virtually unknown. Although Stewart[58] found that patients with a positive delayed hypersensitivity response to the intradermal injection of their own tumour had poorer survival rates than those who failed to react, this has not been confirmed. Roberts has reported that recurrence rates in patients with primary breast cancer who react to their own tumour are the same as in those who fail to do so.

EXTENT OF DISEASE
AND DELAY IN TREATMENT

Extent of disease

The more extensive the disease at the time of primary treatment, the worse is the prognosis. Those criteria which place a tumour in the T3 or T4 category (see page 9) are also grave signs of incurable disease. One which has been particularly studied in several recent reports is tumour size; the larger the tumour, the worse its prognosis[59].

Disseminated disease also heralds a fatal outcome. Routine methods of demonstrating this at the time of primary treatment are relatively inaccurate, and many patients regarded as being free from metastases, already have occult dissemination. This will be further discussed below.

Of particular importance is the influence of axillary node involvement, long known to be associated with a reduction in 5-year survival rates from approximately 70 to 30%. The studies of Cutler and his associates[39] and of Champion and Wallace[60], have shown that the influence of this dominates other factors such as the size of the tumour, the occurrence of lymphocytic infiltration and of sinus histiocytosis in regional nodes. As 75% of the lymph draining the breast passes through the axillary nodes, their involvement is probably the most accurate index of spread of tumour beyond the breast, and therefore of its incurability.

It should be noted that one cannot assume that the prognosis of patients with axillary node involvement is unfavourable because the axillary nodes are involved. It is equally feasible that tumours with an inherently unfavourable prognosis may be more likely to spread early to regional nodes.

The prognostic effect of axillary node metastases is not an all-or-none phenomenon. The number of nodes involved and the extent of that involvement are also important.

Number

In 1961, Pickren[61], from a study of 199 consecutive radical mastectomy specimens, reported a relationship between the number of nodes involved and 5-year survival rates which was almost linear. More recent reports suggest that there may be a cut-off point above which involvement carries a particularly poor prognosis. This is usually defined as 3–4 nodes. According to the findings of Auchincloss[62], involvement of the axillary nodes above the lower border of the pectoralis minor muscle indicates incurable disease.

The curability of those with only a few nodes involved is not well defined. In this situation, other factors may be particularly important. It was reported by Cutler et al.[39], that provided one favourable factor (a small tumour, sinus histiocytosis in regional nodes, or a favourable nuclear grade) is also present the prognosis of patients with less than $\frac{1}{3}$ of the axillary nodes involved is the same as in that with none.

The definition of axillary node involvement is highly inaccurate. It is well recognised that clinical palpability is a poor guide to tumour involvement. Less well recognised is the considerable error also associated with routine pathological examination of the axillary contents. Meticulous examination of removed axillary nodes including serial sections have been carried out in 2 studies[61,63]. These included 81 patients treated by radical mastectomy in which routine pathological examination had been reported as showing no evidence of axillary node involvement; unsuspected cancer was detected in 21 (26%).

Approximately 60% of radical mastectomy specimens contain nodes which on routine examination are involved by tumour. If one adds the error uncovered by the above 2 studies, a more likely estimate of axillary node involvement would be 75%; a figure curiously similar to that of the known incurability rate of primary cancer of the breast.

Extent
The extent of nodal involvement is also related to prognosis. Heavy infiltration of nodes with local fixation (N2) is a grave sign. Conversely the prognosis of patients with "occult" axillary metastases (discovered only on serial section) is better than that of those with overt involvement[61]. It is unknown whether all microscopic foci of tumour cells in the sinusoids of regional nodes flourish.

The influence of delay
It is difficult to prove that delay in seeking treatment for cancer

of the breast materially worsens its prognosis. Studies which relate the interval between the onset of the disease and first treatment to the duration of survival are confusing. In one study of 470 patients treated by radical mastectomy, Bloom[38] found that those whose treatment had been delayed for an average time of 12 months survived as long as those treated within 3 months of the onset of their disease.

There is an obvious paradox. Patients can survive long periods of time without treatment only if their tumours are biologically favourable. Thus they represent a small group of survivors from a population from which those women with tumours of high malignant potential have been eliminated by inoperability or death.

When the inherent malignancy of a tumour is defined by histological grading, a relationship between delay in seeking treatment and survival can be uncovered. In Bloom's series of 1141 patients, rapidly growing tumours of undifferentiated type were, as expected, seen more frequently in those seeking treatment early than in those with a long history. However, when tumour grade was correlated with the extent of the disease at the time of initial treatment and with the length of history, it was found that within each group of tumours of a specified histological grade, delay in treatment increased the incidence of late cases.

Clear statistical evidence of the influence of delay on the results of treatment will come from the New York trial of screening for breast cancer[64]. Over 60 000 women of 40 to 64 years of age have been included. One half were allocated randomly to a screened group in which clinical examination and mammography were performed on entry and at yearly intervals for 3 years; the others were placed in a control group receiving only their usual medical care.

Preliminary results indicate that detection of cancer by screening has reduced the incidence of axillary node involvement and 5-year fatality rates[65]. This was particularly striking in those whose tumours were discovered mammographically before they were clinically palpable. As bringing forward the date of treatment on a fixed time scale will automatically confer an advantage in survival time, a "lead time" of 1 year was included in the survival statistics of the screened group. More time is required to determine if this gives sufficient compensation.

Current trends

These various facts suggest that local therapy is only one factor, and a relatively small one, in determining the curability of cancer of the breast. Of much greater importance is the extent of the disease when the patient first is seen, and to an extent still undefined, the presence or absence of certain biological factors. The impact of these on current trends in the management of the disease will now be considered.

DEFINITION AND EXTENT OF DISEASE

One important trend is to define in much greater detail the extent of the disease before treatment is planned. As this may involve costly and time-consuming studies, it is essential first to make an accurate diagnosis of the disease; methods of doing so are under study.

Although there are still some who believe that clinical examination is adequate, this is far from the case. The increasing recognition of early cancers, in which the only abnormal clinical sign may be a small area of thickening or altered texture of breast tissue makes the likely error of clinical diagnosis greater. In our clinic, despite considerable experience, our error is still 20%.

Mammography has now earned a rightful place as a complement to clinical examination. The study carried out by Stewart et al.[66] in Cardiff is typical of many others. As a sole method of examination its accuracy exceeded that of clinical examination; when both were used together in a complementary way, the accuracy of diagnosis of cancer was 97%.

Although particularly valuable in those patients in whom the clinical signs are equivocal, for example, in the large fatty breast, mammography can also give valuable confirmatory evidence in those with typical clinical features. A spiculated opacity containing punctate calcifications, and associated with altered trabeculation of the breast or skin thickening, can only be a cancer. Mammography also will detect multiple and bilateral tumours.

Xeromammography, in which a xerographic plate is used instead of an X-ray film is a recent development. The plate consists of a sheet of aluminium coated with particles of selenium which bear an electrostatic charge. Following exposure to X-rays, these charged particles form a pattern which represents the image of the breast. This is developed by dusting the plate with coloured talc, the particles of which bear an opposite charge and so adhere to the selenium. As all edges and interfaces are exaggerated by this technique, pathological lesions may be demonstrated more effectively, particularly in the dense glandular breast.

Thermography, by which the pattern of infra-red radiation from the skin of the breast is recorded, is as yet much less accurate. In our study of the accuracy of methods of detecting breast cancer, the best accuracy achieved by thermography was 68%[67].

None of these methods gives a definitive histological diagnosis. The advantages of achieving this before operation are obvious. Not only does it help restrict the need for complex studies to patients with proved diagnosis, but one can proceed to mastectomy without excision biopsy and frozen section examination of the tumour. No matter how carefully this is done, vascular and lymphatic channels in the breast will be opened up, a practice we do not condone for cancer at other sites.

Methods to achieve pre-operative histology are also being evaluated. Drill biopsy, by which a cannula revolving at 20 000 rpm is used to remove a small core of tumour, was 98% accurate[68] in the diagnosis of 281 confirmed cases.

An alternative is needle aspiration biopsy. It can easily be performed with a disposable syringe and No. 1 needle. A small drop of juice is withdrawn from the tumour, expressed onto a slide, stained and examined. The accuracy in experienced hands is high[69,70], but the need of cytological interpretation has prevented wide use of the method.

This apart, needle aspiration is now used with increasing frequency to differentiate cystic from solid lesions of the breast. Aspiration of a cyst is safe therapy, provided certain precautions are taken. In our clinic these include mammography, cytology of cyst fluid, and careful re-assessment of the patient for a residual mass or refilling of the cyst.

INVESTIGATING LUMP

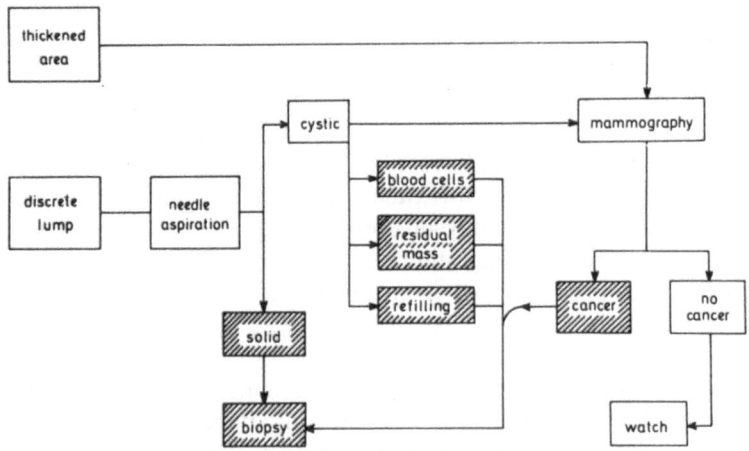

Figure 1.2   Flow diagram of diagnostic procedure used in our breast clinic.

The order in which these various investigations are done will depend on their availability. The flow chart currently used by us is shown in Figure 1.2.

ASSESSMENT OF EXTENT

Clinical staging of breast cancer has 2 main fallacies which affect the management of the disease. One is its reliance on palpability as indicating axillary node involvement; another is its failure to detect occult metastatic deposits.

Axillary nodes

The report by McNair and Dudley[71] first stressed the extent of the observer error of palpation of axillary nodes. Several studies of radical mastectomy specimens have demonstrated an equal error between clinical palpability and histological evidence of tumour involvement. That of Wallace and Champion[72], from this department, is typical. In a study of 174 radical mastectomy specimens, they found evidence of histological invasion by tumour of 45% of palpable and 26% of impalpable nodes. The only certain method of defining axillary node involvement is by histology; yet as discussed above, this also has a considerable error. To be exact serial sections of the nodes are required.

Although the differentiation between Stage 1 and 2 cancer is not too important if the method of primary treatment involves resection of the axillary nodes, it is critical where this includes preservation of the nodes or their treatment by radiotherapy. Otherwise one cannot define with certainty those patients who have axillary node involvement. This could be essential information for their future management. In our experience, the histology of the pectoral nodes, which can be removed without breaching the axilla, is a possible compromise which has proved more accurate than clinical assessment[73].

Occult metastatic disease

The second fallacy of clinical staging is its inability to detect occult metastatic or residual disease. In our experience and that of Galasko[74], routine radiological and biochemical investigations at the time of primary treatment reveal unsuspected metastatic disease in less than 5% of patients with operable Stage 1 and 2 breast cancer. Yet the true incidence of residual cancer must approach 70%. Methods to uncover occult deposits are an essential development.

(i) Lymph node. It is well known that when the axillary nodes are involved histologically, spread to other nodal areas is common. In our series of 50 consecutive cases of operable breast cancer in which we routinely biopsied the supraclavicular and internal mammary nodes, unsuspected deposits were discovered in 7. Despite the further plea by Johnstone[75] that routine biopsy of apical axillary and internal mammary nodes should precede mastectomy, realisation that involvement of any axillary nodes *per se* indicates disease which has a high incurability rate is unlikely to further the practice. It should again be stressed that the prime significance of lymphatic involvement may be as an indicator of disseminated disease.

(ii) Bones. Radiology is a poor method of detecting small foci of metastatic cancer. In a vertebral body a lesion must be 1.5 cm in diameter before it is visible. Skeletal scintiscanning is more discriminating and was reported by Galasko[76] to reveal unsuspected metastatic deposits in 12 of 50 patients with operable cancer of the breast whose X-rays were normal. Eleven of these developed radiological lesions within 4 years.

The principle underlying this method is the avidity for calcium shown by the reparative osteoid reaction around a metastatic deposit. Radioactive compounds of similar biological properties behave similarly and concentrations of ^{87}Sr, ^{18}F, or complexes of technecium-99m and synthetic phosphates can be detected either by rectilinear scanning or gamma scintigraphy.

Before using these refined methods of search, it is important to confirm their validity. In a recent retrospective study of 162 scans performed with ^{87m}Sr and a rectilinear scanner, McCormick et al.[77] in Edinburgh, described a rate of false positive scans of 6%, and of false negative of 26%. Although many of the false negative scans could be explained by low density counts, lesions in the pelvic bones and in the lower dorsal spine were particularly difficult to define. The newer complexes of phosphate and technecium are likely to prove superior.

An alternative method of seeking occult metastatic bone disease is by estimates of urinary hydroxyproline. Increased turnover of the large collagen pool in bone enhances the excretion of this amino-acid: a unique constituent of collagen. Some studies have suggested that its increased secretion may even precede scintiscan evidence of metastatic bone disease[78]. Yet considerable variations of excretion have also been reported in patients with bone metastases[79]. Its validity requires to be further assessed.

Routine marrow and bone biopsies have been used in the past to increase the yield of demonstrable metastatic disease. Both are troublesome and in the future likely to be indicated only by positive scans.

(iii) Viscera. Asymptomatic cerebral metastases are difficult to define and brain scans are rarely used in patients with primary cancer of the breast. Most patients have tests of liver function before surgery but those used routinely lack sensitivity. According to Magnum and Powell[80], liver scans are more likely to detect metastases than routine tests of liver function. Alkaline phosphatase isoenzymes and γ glutamyl transpeptidase may give better discrimination in the future. Meantime preoperative liver scans with laparscopic biopsy of those with positive findings is an obvious line of investigation. The accuracy of radiology for the detection of pulmonary metastases has not been superseded.

To many these investigations may appear to be unnecessarily elaborate. Yet unless efforts are made to detect the spread of breast cancer before treatment, we will continue to waste our efforts on local management, instead of considering how best to use systemic therapy. The accurate staging of lymphomas has revolutionised their treatment; the same should apply to solid tumours, such as those of the breast.

CONSERVATIVE LOCAL THERAPY

There is a trend towards more conservative local therapy. This is due to the realisation that occult generalised disease is all too common, a desire to preserve the immunological function of regional lymph nodes, and also to prevent undue morbidity.

There are few comparative studies of the morbidity caused by the various methods used to treat primary cancer of the breast. Only one study used a protocol which was specifically designed for the purpose, and then in a selective group of patients, over 90% of whom had been treated by radical mastectomy[81]. An assessment of morbidity in patients randomly allocated to different treatment groups was made in the Copenhagen trial, but only in respect of arm swelling[10].

In Cardiff, we carried out a study of morbidity in patients randomly allocated within a controlled randomised trial for treatment either by simple mastectomy with selective radiotherapy according to the histology of the pectoral nodes, or by radical mastectomy, followed by post-operative radiotherapy if resected nodes contained tumour. A detailed protocol was used for subjective and objective assessment. This included a home visit to interview the patient's family[95].

It was found that removal of the breast caused anxiety and embarrassment to the majority of women. Diminished arm function and arm swelling were more frequent in patients who had their axillary nodes dissected or irradiated than those in whom they had been left untreated. There was no marked additive effect between radiotherapy and axillary node surgery, except in respect of arm function. This was impaired to the greatest extent in those who had received both forms of treatment. In terms of morbidity there was a real advantage in leaving the axillary contents undisturbed. Simple mastectomy alone was preferable either to radical mastectomy, or to simple mastectomy with radiotherapy. It was also notable that patients tolerated a transverse scar better than one placed obliquely, which could prevent the wearing of low-necked clothes.

Since the original report of Qualheim and Gall[82], 2 other studies of whole sections of breasts containing primary tumours have revealed a surprising incidence of multifocal disease[87,96]. In our study, Stewart et al.[42], using the paper section technique of Gough and Wentworth[84], reported that 38% of 50 breasts removed for the treatment of primary cancer contained more than one deposit of tumour. These findings suggest that treatment must be of the whole breast, either by its surgical removal, or by local excision combined with intensive radiotherapy.

The need to resect the axillary nodes, or to treat them by radiotherapy is less certain. Both on the grounds of preservation of immunological function and of prevention of morbidity, there is good reason to adopt a watching policy in those whose nodes are most likely to be uninvolved. This is being put to the test in 2 controlled trials.

Cancer research campaign trial
The object of this multi-centre trial, instituted at Cambridge and King's College Hospital, is to determine if treatment of patients with clinical Stage 1 and 2 cancers (T1 + 2, N0 + 1, M0) by simple mastectomy and careful follow-up (with treatment of the nodal areas by radiotherapy is subsequently required) gives results equal to those of simple mastectomy followed by routine radiotherapy to skin flaps, axilla and supraclavicular and internal mammary areas[85]. Although only preliminary results have been reported, it would seem that there is no immediate danger in adopting a watching policy as far as the axilla is concerned. In fact the majority of axillary nodes which were palpable at the time of inclusion of the patient into the trial, and which were left untreated, became impalpable within 3 months[86]. As palpability does not indicate metastatic

involvement, this finding cannot be construed as an indication of spontaneous regression of nodes involved by tumour. It may be due to resolution of reactive changes as a result of removal of the diseased breast.

Cardiff trial

The second trial was one which we instituted in Cardiff and St. Mary's Hospital to determine if a policy of selective simple mastectomy based on histological sampling of the pectoral nodes would give results equal to those of a standard radical approach[87]. The main lymphatic drainage of the breast to the axilla passes through these nodes which lie alongside the medial border of the axillary tail of the breast in relation to the lateral thoracic vessels. They can readily be identified when the axillary tail is being dissected during a total (simple) mastectomy and may either be removed with the tail, or dissected out separately for histological examination.

The policy of treatment under trial was a simple mastectomy with adjuvant radiotherapy to the axilla, 4000 rad over 3 weeks, if the histology of these nodes was positive. If involvement of the nodes was not demonstrated, no radiotherapy was given, but a watching policy adopted. Those randomly allocated to the contrast group were treated by a standard radical approach in which in continuity resection of the breast and axillary nodes was performed. Radical post-operative radiotherapy was also given if the axillary nodes were proved to contain tumour.

Although no significant findings in terms of recurrence-free survival are yet available, it is clear that this policy of selective simple mastectomy carries a lower morbidity than a standard radical approach, and that a policy for watching the axilla, based on the histology of the pectoral nodes, is not followed by a worrying incidence of recurrent disease. There is also evidence that pectoral node biopsy is a more accurate guide to axillary node status than clinical palpability[73].

This policy of treatment is being further studied in Edinburgh, where the current orthodox practice of treating breast cancer is by simple mastectomy and routine radiotherapy. The operation to be performed is a simple mastectomy with pectoral node biopsy; those with negative nodes will be randomly allocated either for routine radiotherapy, or for inclusion in a watched group in which no immediate radiotherapy will be given. Its objective is to determine to what extent irradiation of regional nodes which are not involved by tumour is harmful to the patient, either regarding the progress of the disease, or, in terms of unnecessary morbidity.

ADDITIONAL SYSTEMATIC THERAPY

In line with more conservative local therapy, there is also evidence of more radical use of additional systemic therapy as part of the initial treatment of the disease. Its object is to eradicate residual tumour. Although evidence of its value is not yet impressive, there are now several controlled randomised studies in which the treatment of primary disease by orthodox local therapy is being compared with that of orthodox therapy plus additional therapy of various types.

It is important that patients should be selected for inclusion in these trials on the grounds of likely incurability; otherwise one might obscure differences by the inclusion of those patients with more favourable disease. In the Edinburgh trial we intend to include those, who at simple mastectomy have proved involvement of pectoral nodes and those with locally advanced disease (Stage 3) in whom local therapy would only normally be used. These indications are likely to widen when better methods of detecting occult metastatic disease become generally available; one might also justifiably include tumours of primitive nuclear grade and those which were not associated with evidence of immunological activity.

The selection of systemic therapy is not easy. As only about 40% of tumours are hormone-sensitive, endocrine treatment is unlikely to be uniformly beneficial. Its rational use is dependent upon the development of reliable methods of predicting hormone dependence. Most promising are the methods to determine oestrogen receptor protein and other hormone influences on tumour growth *in vitro*.

Immunotherapy is still in its infancy and largely untried in solid tumours. However, it may well be of value, either alone or in combination with other therapy. Possible methods have been reviewed by Woodruff[88].

Meantime reliance is likely to be placed on chemotherapy.

The drug of choice must be of proved value in established disease, yet free from those side effects which might affect normal wellbeing. As it it more likely to be effective when administered in pulse doses over a prolonged period, ease of administration is important. Intensive regimes of multiple chemotherapy such as those described by Cooper[89] are not likely to gain acceptance for the treatment of fit women. Not only do they require hospitalisation of the patient, but they can cause considerable illhealth. A single agent is more likely to prove acceptable, particularly if therapy is to be continued for months or even years.

SPECIAL TYPES OF DISEASE

Some of the factors which have been discussed affect the management of special types of disease. Two factors deserve recognition when considering cancer in *pre-menopausal women*. One is the pill, the other pregnancies. Although there is no evidence that the contraceptive pill influences adversely the risk of developing cancer of the breast, or its subsequent behaviour, most surgeons disallow this form of contraception for the young woman with breast cancer. This advice is probably wise. The reports of Peters[35], which have been described above, indicate that *pregnancy and breast cancer* are not such sinister companions as was once believed. According to her findings, cancer of the breast occurring during the first half of pregnancy should be treated by orthodox means, and the pregnancy allowed to continue. Should the disease be discovered during its second half, the breast should not be treated until the pregnancy has either been terminated, or allowed to go to term. The young woman who has been treated curatively for cancer of the breast need not fear subsequent pregnancies. Although it is probably wise to advise against a pregnancy during the initial 2 years after treatment in which recurrent disease is more likely to occur, it is reasonable to allow this after that time.

There is no need to specify particular forms of treatment for *cancer of the male breast*. This is a rare disease. On account of the small size of the breast it is usually locally advanced when first seen. For this reason a high proportion of cases are initially treated by radiotherapy alone. Orchidectomy has proved effective endocrine surgery for the advanced case; there is every indication to proceed with this should it be suspected that dissemination has occurred.

It is important to suspect *Paget's disease* in any patient with recent excoriation or crusting of the nipple. Mammography may demonstrate the underlying lesion by an opacity or intraduct calcifications; if so, mastectomy should be proceeded with. If no lesion is seen in the breast, a biopsy of the nipple is mandatory; if this is positive, the patient should be treated by mastectomy. In this disease and in intraduct cancer presenting in other ways, a local (simple) mastectomy with pectoral node biopsy is the most that need be done.

Lobular carcinoma in which the tumour arises from acinar as opposed to duct epithelium, is rare and usually described as an incidental histological finding in biopsies for fibrocystic disease. In the literature there has been confusion between this condition and what we term "epitheliosis". If non-invasive, wide local excision is adequate treatment; if invasive, mastectomy is indicated. Bilateral disease is particularly common.

In view of their greater likelihood to metastasise to internal mammary nodes, *medial tumours* also present a problem. There is justification for irradiating the internal mammary chain as part of primary therapy, but no clear evidence that this will aid cure. It is our current practice to biopsy the second and/or third internal mammary nodes and to base treatment on the histological findings.

A problem which is still unclear is *bilaterality*. A patient with cancer of the breast is 3–4 times more likely to develop a tumour of the opposite breast than a normal woman of the same age[90]. The annual incidence of involvement has been calculated to be 6–7 cases per year per 1000 at risk[91]. Approximately half of all second tumours are metastatic.

Bilateral cancer is particularly common in women under 50 years of age if the first tumour be multiple or if it be an intraduct or invasive lobular carcinoma. Mammography of the second breast at the time of initial treatment is therefore important. It is advised that routine biopsy of the upper outer quadrant of the opposite breast or even mastectomy of the second breast be carried out on those with intraduct or invasive cancer.

Mammography also may be used to follow up the second breast after initial treatment and will detect tumours before they are clinically palpable.

Little attention has been paid to the effect of *early diagnosis* on the management of the disease. Yet the New York study referred to above, suggests that this may have worthwhile rewards. Screening programmes are costly, and unlikely ever to be applicable to the whole female population; the definition of high risk groups is therefore important.

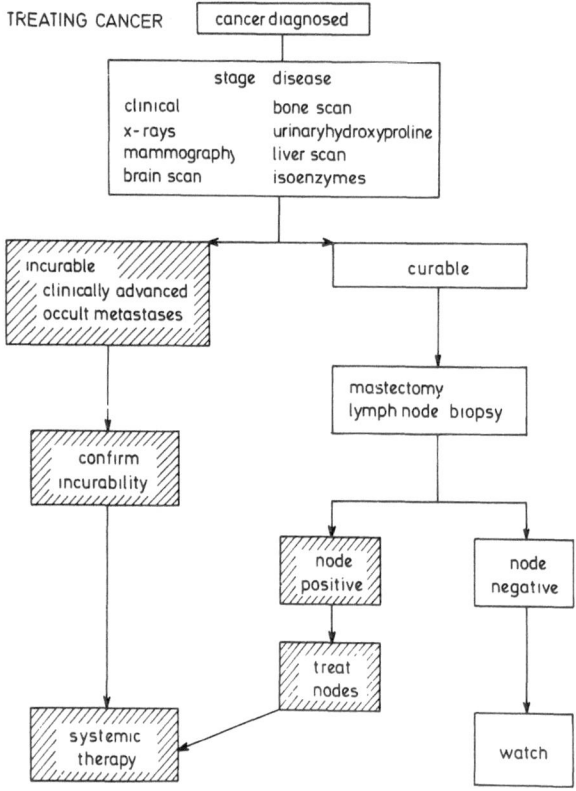

Figure 1.3   Flow diagram of policy of treatment of primary breast cancer based on the principles documented in this chapter

Conclusions

It is obvious that it is not yet possible to formulate clear indications for the management of cancer of the breast with hope of cure. These have become confused and irrational, mainly on account of the preoccupation of surgeons and radiotherapists with methods of local therapy; which in at least 70% of patients with so called "curable" and "operable" disease are ineffective. Early and accurate diagnosis, and the use of more effective methods of detecting dissemination are essential prerequisites of rational therapy. The result will be the direction of treatment to sites of proved involvement resulting in more conservative local and more radical systemic therapy.

An order of procedure according to the policies which have been discussed is given in Figure 1.3. This includes a careful primary search for evidence of metastatic disease before initial therapy is planned, and for a secondary division according to the state of the lymph nodes in the axilla. Cases would be treated by simple mastectomy alone, by simple mastectomy with treatment of regional nodes by resection or radiotherapy, and by systemic therapy according to the stage of the disease. Within any such policy careful watching of untreated areas is essential.

The type of systemic therapy to be employed should be based on those factors which affect the prognosis of the disease and may well vary according to the endocrine and immune characteristics of the tumour. Proof that a policy of this type will cure a larger number of patients is not available and can come only from the institution of controlled clinical trials. It is the duty of all who treat the disease to participate.

Acknowledgements

The construction of an opinion is seldom personal.

I am greatly indebted to those with whom I have discussed, at length, some of the principles set out in this chapter; particularly, Dr A. O. Langlands, Dr Maureen Roberts, Miss Helen Stewart and Miss Elizabeth Cant. I also am grateful to Mrs. Janet Wake for her secretarial help.

REFERENCES

1. Forrest, A. P. M. (1969. Breast cancer symposium: points in the practical management of breast cancer. *Brit. J. Surg.*, **56**, 782

2. Nemoto, T. (1973). Treatment of early breast cancer. *New York St. J. Med.*, **73**, 1901

3. Easson, E. C. and Russell, M. H. (1968). *The Curability of Cancer in Various Sites.* London, Pitman

4. Bloom, H. J. G. (1968). Survival of women with untreated breast cancer — past and present. *Prognostic Factors in Breast Cancer.* Edited by A. P. M. Forrest and P. B. Kunkler, p. 3. Edinburgh and London: Livingstone

5. Auchincloss, H. (1958). The nature of local recurrence following radical mastectomy. *Cancer*, **7**, 11, 611

6. Collins, V. P. (1956). Breast cancer: influence of treatment that fails to cure. *Cancer*, **9**, 1177

7. Tough, I. C. K. (1966). The significance of recurrence in breast cancer. *Brit. J. Surg.*, **53**, 897

8. Bruce, J., Carter, D. C. and Fraser, J. (1970). Patterns of recurrent disease in breast cancer. *Lancet*, **i**, 433

9. Taylor, G. W. and Nathanson, I. T. (1942). *Lymph Node Metastases.* New York: Oxford University Press

10. Kaae, S. and Johansen, H. (1968). Simple versus radical mastectomy for primary breast cancer. *Prognostic Factors in Breast Cancer.* Edited by A. P. M. Forrest and P. B. Kunkler, p. 93. Edinburgh and London: Livingstone

11. Brinkley, D. M. and Haybittle, J. L. (1966). Treatment of stage II carcinoma of the female breast. *Lancet*, **ii**, 291

12. Bruce, J. (1971). Operable cancer of the breast: a controlled clinical trial. *Cancer*, **28**, 1443

13. Paterson, R. and Russell, M. H. (1959). Clinical trials in malignant disease part III. Breast cancer: evaluation of post-operative radiotherapy. *J. Fac. Radiol.*, **10**, 175

14. Easson, E. C. (1968). Post-operative radiotherapy in breast cancer. *Prognostic Factors in Breast Cancer.* Edited by A. P. M. Forrest and P. B. Kunkler, p. 118. Edinburgh and London: Livingstone

15. Fisher, B. (1971). Status of adjuvant therapy: results of the national surgical adjuvant breast project studies on oophorectomy (post-operative radiation therapy and chemotherapy), *Cancer*, **28**, 1654

16. Atkins, H., Hayward, J. L., Klugman, D. J. and Wayte, A. B. (1972). Treatment of early breast cancer: a report after ten years of a clinical trial. *Brit. Med. J.*, **2**, 423

17. Watson, T. A., Bond, A. F. and Phillips, A. J. (1963). Swelling and disfunction of the upper limb following radical mastectomy. *Surg. Gynaec. Obstet.*, **116**, 99

18. Gray, J. H. (1939). The relation of lymphatic vessels to the spread of cancer. *Brit. J. Surg.*, **26**, 462

19. Turner-Warwick, R. T. (1959). The lymphatics of the breast. *Brit. J. Surg.*, **46**, 574

20. Patey, D. H. and Dyson, W. H. (1948). Prognosis of carcinoma of the breast in relation to type of operation performed. *Brit. J. Cancer*, **2**, 7

21. Kendall, B. E., Arthur, J. F. and Patey, D. H. (1963). Lymphangiography in carcinoma of the breast. A comparison of clinical radiological and pathological findings in axillary lymph nodes. *Cancer*, **16**, 1233

22. Cole, M. P. (1968). Suppression of ovarian function in primary cancer of the breast. *Prognostic Factors in Breast Cancer*. Edited by A. P. M. Forrest and P. B. Kunkler, p. 146. Edinburgh and London: Livingstone

23. Nissen-Meyer, R. (1968). Suppression of ovarian function in primary cancer of the breast. *Prognostic Factors in Breast Cancer*. Edited by A. P. M. Forrest and P. B. Kunkler, p. 139. Edinburgh and London: Livingstone

24. Patey, D. H. (1960). Prophylactic oophorectomy and adrenalectomy in carcinoma of the breast. *Brit. J. Cancer*, **14**, 457

25. Dao, T. L., Nemoto, T. and Chamberlain, A. (1973). Adrenalectomy with radical mastectomy in the treatment of high risk breast cancer. (To be published)

26. Meakin, J. W., Allt, W. E. C., Beale, F. A., Brown, T. C., Clark, R. M., Fitzpatrick, P. J., Hopkins, N. V., Jenkin, R. D. T., Bulbrook, T. D. and Hayward, J. L. (1968). Preliminary report of two studies of adjuvant treatment of primary breast cancer. *Prognostic Factors in Breast Cancer*. Edited by A. P. M. Forrest and P. B. Kunkler, p. 157. Edinburgh and London: Livingstone

27. Lyons, A. R. (1968). Thyroid hormones and breast cancer. *Prognostic Factors in Breast Cancer*. Edited by A. P. M. Forrest and P. B. Kunkler, p. 164. Edinburgh and London: Livingstone

28. Riache, K., Beradt, H. and Prahl, B. (1972). Continuous post-operative treatment with cyclophosphamide in breast carcinoma — a randomised clinical study. *Arch. Geschwurlst Fursch.*, **40**, 349

29. Nissen-Meyer, R., Kjellgren, K. and Mansson, A. (1971). Preliminary report from the Scandinavian adjuvant chemotherapy study group. *Cancer Chemotherapy Report*, **55**, 561

30. Wynder, E. L. (1968). Current concepts of the aetiology of breast cancer. *Prognostic Factors in Breast Cancer*. Edited by A. P. M. Forrest and P. B. Kunkler, p. 32. Edinburgh and London: Livingstone

31. MacMahon, B., List, N. D. and Eisenberg, H. (1968). Relationship of survival of breast cancer patients to parity and menopausal status. *Prognostic Factors in Breast Cancer*. Edited by A. P. M. Forrest and P. B. Kunkler, p. 56. Edinburgh and London: Livingstone

32. MacMahon, B., Cole, P. and Brown, J. (1973). Aetiology of hormones in breast cancer: a review. *J. Nat. Canc. Inst.*, **50**, 21

33. Lowe, C. R. and MacMahon, B. (1970). Breast cancer and reproductive history of women in South Wales. *Lancet*, **i**, 153

34. MacKay, E. N. and Sellers, A. H. (1965). Breast cancer at the Ontario Cancer Clinics 1938–1956. A statistical review. Ontario medical statistics branch (Ontario Department of Health)

35. Peters, M. V. (1968). The effect of pregnancy in breast cancer. *Prognostic Factors in Breast Cancer*. Edited by A. P. M. Forrest and P. B. Kunkler, p. 65. Edinburgh and London: Livingstone

36. Hayward, J. L. and Bulbrook, R. D. (1968). Urinary steroids and prognosis in breast cancer. *Prognostic Factors in Breast Cancer*. Edited by A. P. M. Forrest and P. B. Kunkler, p. 383. Edinburgh and London: Livingstone

37. Bloom, H. J. G. and Richardson, W. W. (1957). Histological grading and prognosis in breast cancer. A study of 1409 cases of which 359 have been followed for 15 years. *Brit. J. Cancer*, **11**, 359

38. Bloom, H. J. G. (1965). The influence of delay on the natural history and prognosis of breast cancer. A study of cases followed for 5–20 years. *Brit. J. Cancer*, **19**, 228

39. Cutler, S. J., Black, M. M., Mork, T., Harvell, S. and Freeman, C. (1969). Further observations on prognostic factors in cancer of the female breast. *Cancer*, **24**, 653

40. Gorski, C. M., Niepolomska, W., Nowak, K., Gebbel, B., Plewa, T., Pysz, H. and Adamus, J. (1968). Clinical evaluation and pathological grading in relation to other prognostic factors. *Prognostic Factors in Breast Cancer*. Edited by A. P. M. Forrest and P. B. Kunkler, p. 309. Edinburgh and London: Livingstone

41. Champion, H. R. and Wallace, I. W. J. (1971). Breast cancer grading. *Brit. J. Cancer*, **25**, 441

42. Stewart, H. J., Williams, W. J., Apsimon, H. T., Gravelle, I. H. and Forrest, A. P. M. (1968). The relationship of tumour contour to other prognostic factors in breast cancer. *Prognostic Factors in Breast Cancer*. Edited by A. P. M. Forrest and P. B. Kunkler, p. 301. Edinburgh and London: Livingstone

43. Ingleby, H. and Gershon-Cohen, J. (1960). Comparative anatomy, pathology and roentgenology of the breast, p. 359. Philadelphia: University of Pennsylvania Press

44. Lane, N., Goskel, H., Salerno, R. A. and Haagensan, C. D. (1961). Clinico-pathologic analysis of the surgical curability of breast cancer. *Ann. Surg.*, **153**, 483

45. Shivas, A. A. and Douglas, J. G. (1973). The prognostic significance of elastosis in breast carcinoma. *J. Royal College Surg. Ed.*, **17**, 315

46. Black, M. M., Opler, S. R. and Speer, F. D. (1955). Survival in breast cancer cases in relation to the structure of the primary tumour and regional lymph nodes. *Surg. Gynec. Obst.*, **100**, 543

47. Berg, J. W. (1962). Active host resistance to breast cancer. *Acta Union Contra Cancer*, **18**, 854

48. Hamlin, E. (1968). Possible host resistance in carcinoma of the breast: a histological study. *Brit. J. Cancer*, **22**, 383

49. Stewart, T. H. M. (1969). The presence of delayed hypersensitivity reaction in patients towards cellular extracts of their malignant tumours. *Cancer*, **23**, 1380.

50. Roberts, M. M., Bass, E. M., Skoenson, A. and Wallace, I. W. J. (1973). Local immunoglobulin production in breast cancer *Brit. J. Cancer*, **27**, 269

51. Moore, O. S. and Foote, F. W. (1949). The relatively favourable prognosis of medullary carcinoma of the breast. *Cancer*, **2**, 635

52. Bloom, H. J. C. (1970). Host resistance and survival in carcinoma of the breast: a study of 104 cases of medullary carcinoma in a series of 1411 cases of breast cancer followed for 20 years. *Brit. Med. J.*, **3**, 181

53. Cutler, S. J. (1968). The prognosis of treated cancer of the breast. *Prognostic Factors in Breast Cancer*. Edited by A. P. M. Forrest and P. B. Kunkler, p. 20. Edinburgh and London: Livingstone

54. Black, M. M., Kerpe, S. and Speer, F. D. (1953). Lymph node structure in patients with breast cancer. *Amer. J. Path.*, **29**, 505

55. Daoud, E. S. (1964). Prognostic significance of sinus histiocytosis in regional lymph nodes and of the local presence of round cells in human cancer. Ph.D. thesis, University of Wales

56. Good, R. A. (1973). Perspectives in Oncology. Clark lecture given to Edinburgh Pathological Club

57. Hughes, L. E. and MacKay, W. D. (1965). Suppression of tuberculin response in malignant disease. *Brit. Med. J.*, **2**, 1346

58. Stewart, T. H. M. and Orizaga, M. (1971). The presence of delayed hypersensitivity reactions in patients towards cellular extract of their tumours. III: The frequency, duration and cross reactivity of this phenomenon in patients with breast cancer and its correlation with survival. *Cancer*, **28**, 1472

59. Cutler, S. J. (1966). The value of general survival data in clinical evaluation in breast cancer, p. 215. *Clinical Evaluation in Breast Cancer*. Edited by J. L. Hayward and R. D. Bulbrook. Academic Press: New York

60. Champion, H. R., Wallace, I. W. J. and Prescott, R. J. (1972). Histology in breast cancer prognosis. *Brit. J. Cancer*, **26**, 129

61. Pickren, J. W. (1961). Significance of occult metastases. *Cancer*, **14**, 1266

62. Auchincloss, H. (1963). Significance and location and number of axillary metastases in carcinoma of the breast. A justification for a conservative operation. *Ann. Surg.*, **158**, 37

63. Saphir, O. and Amronin, G. D. (1948). Obscure axillary lymph node metastases in carcinoma of the breast. *Cancer*, **1**, 238

64. Strax, P., Venet, L., Shapiro, S. and Gross, S. (1967). Mammography and clinical examination in mass screening for cancer of the breast. *Cancer*, **20**, 2184

65. Strax, P. (1974). Personal communication

66. Stewart, H. J., Gravelle, I. H. and Apsimon, H. J. (1969). Five years experience with mammography. *Brit. J. Surg.*, **56**, 341

67. Furnival, I. G., Stewart, H. J., Weddell, J. M., Dovey, P., Gravelle, I. H., Evans, K. T. and Forrest, A. P. M. (1970). Accuracy of screening methods for the diagnosis of breast disease. *Brit. Med. J.*, **2**, 461

68. Nathan, B. E., Burn, J. H. and Doyle, F. H. (1972). An evaluation of mammography in breast clinics. *Clin. Radiol.*, **23**, 87

69. Franzen, S. and Zajicek, J. (1968). Aspiration biopsy in diagnosis of palpable lesions of the breast. Critical review of 3479 cross section biopsies. *Acta Radiol. Scand.*, **7**, 241

70. Webb, A. J. (1970). The diagnostic cytology of breast carcinoma. *Brit. J. Surg.*, **57**, 259

71. McNair, T. J. and Dudley, H. A. F. (1960). Axillary lymph nodes in patients with breast carcinoma. *Lancet*, **i**, 713

72. Wallace, I. W. J. and Champion, H. R. (1972). Axillary lymph nodes in breast cancer. *Lancet*, **i**, 217

73. Roberts, M. M., Forrest, A. P. M., Blumgart, L. H., Campbell, H. and eight other contributors (1973). Simple versus radical mastectomy. *Lancet*, **ii**, 1073

74. Galasko, C. S. B. (1972). Skeletal metastases and mammary cancer. *Ann. Roy. Coll. Surg. Eng.*, **50**, 3

75. Johnstone, F. R. C. (1972). Results of treatment of carcinoma of the breast based on pathological staging. *Surg. Gynec. Obst.*, **134**, 211

76. Galasko, C. S. B. (1969). The detection of skeletal metastases from mammary cancer by gamma camera scintigraphy. *Brit. J. Surg.*, **56**, 757

77. McCormick, J. StC., Aldrich, J. E., Summerling, M. D. (1974). The value of scintigraphy in the detection of skeletal metastases from mammary cancer in a review of 162 strontium-87m bone scans. (in press)

78. Cuschieri, A. and Felgate, R. A. (1972). Urinary hydroxyproline excretions in carcinoma of the breast. *Brit. J. Exp. Surg.*, **53**, 237
79. Ditzel, J., Jordal, R. and Riskaer, N. (1968). Total urinary hydroxyproline excretion before and after hypophysectomy in patients with bone metastases from breast carcinoma. *Acta Endocr.*, **59**, 353
80. Mangum, J. F. and Powell, M. R. (1973). Liver scintophotography as an index for liver abnormality' *J. Int. Med.*, **14**, 484
81. Eisenberg, H. S. and Goldenberg, I. S. (1966). A measurement of quality of survival of breast cancer patients. *Clinical Evaluation in Breast Cancer.* Edited by J. L. Hayward and R. D. Bulbrook. Academic Press: London and New York
82. Qualheim, R. E. and Gall, E. A. (1957). Breast carcinoma with multiple sites of origin. *Cancer*, **10**, 460
83. Gallagher, H. S. and Martin, J. E. (1969). The study of mammary carcinoma by mammography and whole organ sectioning. *Cancer*, **23**, 855
84. Gough, J. and Wentworth, J. E. (1960). Thin sections of entire organs mounted on paper. *Advances in pathology*, 7th edition, p. 80. Edited by C. V. Harrison. Churchill: London
85. Baum, M., Edwards, M. H. and Margarey, C. J. (1972). Organisation of clinical trials on a national scale. Management of early cancer of the breast. *Brit. Med. J.*, **4**, 476
86. Edwards, M. H., Baum, M. and Margarey, C. J. (1972). Regression of axillary lymph nodes in cancer of the breast. *Brit. J. Surg.*, **59**, 776
87. Forrest, A. P. M., Gleave, E. N., Roberts, M. M., Henk, J. M. and Gravelle, I. H. (1970). A controlled trial of conservative treatment for early breast cancer. *Proc. Roy. Soc. Med.*, **63**, 107
88. Woodruff, M. F. A. (1972). Residual cancer. Harvey lectures, series 66, p. 161. New York
89. Cooper, R. G. (1969). Combination chemotherapy in hormone resistant breast cancer. *Proc. Amer. Assoc. Cancer Res.*, **10**, 15
90. Kilgore, A. R. (1921). The incidence of cancer of the second breast. *J. Amer. Med. Assoc.*, **77**, 454
91. Robbins, G. F. and Berg, J. W. (1964). Bilateral primary breast cancers. A prospective clinicopathological study. *Cancer*, **17**, 1501
92. Brimkley, D. and Haybittle, J. L.'(1968). A 15-year follow-up study of patients treated for cancer of the breast. *Brit. J. Radiol.*, **41**, 215
93. Roberts, M. M. (1974). Cellular immunity in human breast cancer. M.D. thesis, University of Wales.
94. Roberts, M. M. (1974). Lymphocyte function in breast cancer. *Europe. J. Surg. Res.*, (in press)
95. Roberts, M. M., Furnival, I. G. and Forrest, A. P. M. (1972). The morbidity of mastectomy. *Brit. J. Surg.*, **59**, 301
96. Stewart, H. J. Unpublished data

2

Techniques of surgical treatment

R. S. Handley

*"Our fathers thought themselves a great deal nearer to per-
fection than we have found them to be; and I am much mistaken if our successors do not, in more instances than one,
wonder both at our inattention and our ignorance".* Percival
Pott, circa 1775 (quoted by Miss Jessie Dobson[1]).

Surgical techniques for the treatment of breast cancer range
from the ultra conservative to the ultra radical, and no
unanimous message has emerged to show which is the best.
Many controlled trials are now proceeding to try to settle this
point. There is in any case not one "best" method of treatment
because cases vary so greatly in the extent of their disease when
they present, in their general health and in the malignancy of
their tumours, that treatment which is appropriate in one
patient may be contraindicated in the next.

    Whatever technique any individual surgeon adopts, he can
find in the literature respected authority to support him. This
divergence of opinion after a hundred years of recognisably
rational therapy, must support the opinion, expressed by
Sir Hedley Atkins in 1953, that the method of treatment makes
a difference to the end result in only some 10% of patients. To
consider only the end result however is to disregard an important
part of the equation, namely the post-operative quality of a
patient's life (which is a much more difficult thing to measure).
To those of us who believe that the quality of life is as important,
if not more important, than its quantity, this consideration adds
a disturbing element to our thinking.

Pathological considerations

To formulate any reasonable hypothesis as to how breast cancer
is likely to be most successfully treated, one must consider, at

the risk of some repetition, the pathological processes at work in the dissemination of malignant disease — processes which we do not even now fully understand.

So far as the breast is concerned, direct infiltration poses no serious obstacle to modern surgery and can be dismissed. It is the spread of malignant cells by the blood vessels and the lymphatics which lie at the root of the problem, coupled with the equally important factors of tumour malignancy and host resistance.

BLOOD SPREAD

To take first the dissemination of cancer cells via the blood vessels, it seems that this is much more important than was believed even 25 years ago. It was at one time thought that it was a late event, but it now seems likely that malignant cells may circulate in the blood at a very early stage and often before a breast tumour is clinically apparent. My own reasons for supposing this to be so are as follows: firstly we see patients who, despite histological evidence that there is no lymph node metastasis or other evidence of spread outside the breast die of recurrences within a year or two. Secondly it seems curious that all the reports which I have seen of investigations into the presence of circulating cancer cells in the blood of breast cancer patients have shown some — though widely differing — percentages of positive results. When one recollects that these investigations are mostly based on a 10 ml sample of blood, taken perhaps in $\frac{1}{2}$ min, one cannot help thinking that if the whole blood volume could somehow be monitored all the time, every case would be positive. Thirdly, there is accumulating evidence that there are lympho–venous anastomoses in lymph nodes and that all lymph does not return to the blood via the thoracic duct and the other main lymphatic channels. The work of Fisher and Fisher[2] on the behaviour of the popliteal lymph node of the rabbit, when the node receives isotope-tagged experimental tumour cells, is particularly interesting in this connection. Fourthly, Galasko's demonstration, by the use of F 18 and the γ camera, that 12 of his 50 early breast cancer patients had bony metastases, unrevealed by conventional radiology, adds further confirmation.

Fortunately there is evidence that the discovery of a tumour cell in the blood is not synonymous with a successful metastasis. These cells suffer an enormous — and with luck a total — mortality. Roberts and his colleagues[4] have shown, in a follow-up of 749 cases who had been investigated for the presence of breast cancer cells in the blood, that the prognosis was no different whether such cells had been demonstrated or not.

LYMPHATIC SPREAD
For the surgeon the lymphatic paths of malignant spread are perhaps even more important than the blood vessels, because he may be able to do something about them. It is only in the last 25 years that it has been generally recognised that the lymphatic drainage of the breast is not only to the axillary lymph nodes. In 534 cases in which the lymph nodes were thought not to be invaded (clinical Stage 1) I found[5] that 15% had invasion of the internal mammary lymph nodes; and if Stages 1 and 2 were added together, the 842 patients, deemed to be "operable", showed a 21% invasion rate of these nodes. Until recently no notice was taken (with a few exceptions) either by surgeons or radiotherapists, of the internal mammary lymph nodes, though they constituted no small loophole in the efficacy of treatment.

Though the axillary and the internal mammary systems are the principal lymphatic exits from the breast, there are other minor channels which run straight into the intercostal spaces to discharge into nodes lying on the necks of the ribs.

OTHER PATHOLOGICAL CONSIDERATIONS
There are 3 other pathological considerations which must affect the choice of therapeutic techniques.
(i) Multifocal carcinoma. The frequency with which breast cancer arises as a multifocal process in the breast is still a matter for debate. That it sometimes does so is known to every experienced clinician. Pathological investigation of breasts removed for carcinoma suggest that a multifocal origin is much more frequent than clinical experience would suggest. Thus Qualheim and Gall[6] found a multifocal origin in 54% of the 157 breasts which they examined. This is the highest figure I have encountered, but others, e.g. Muir[7] have pointed out that carcinoma of the breast does not always originate in a single

focus, a view which Cheatle and Cutler had propounded in 1931. The difficulty in judging the frequency with which carcinoma arises in the breast as a multifocal process is to know what pre-malignant and pre-invasive changes in the epithelium are going to progress to invasive carcinoma; and indeed what hyperplastic epithelial changes are pre-malignant. The occurrence of multifocal carcinoma is a fact, but its frequency varies with the individual view of the pathologist in his interpretation of the potential of pathologically hyperplastic epithelium. Gallager and Martin[8] regard this latter as "a non-obligate pre-neoplastic lesion", by which they mean that such areas may progress to an invasive carcinoma or regress to a normal state.

(ii) Tumour malignancy. While histological appraisal of the malignancy of a tumour does not influence most surgeons in the choice of a technique, it is generally agreed that the clinical appearances of an inflammatory carcinoma do contraindicate any form of surgery beyond biopsy.

(iii) Host resistance. This fascinating and intensely difficult aspect of tumour growth has influenced surgeons in their choice of techniques but it is perhaps safe to say that little certain knowledge at present exists to direct the way in which therapy should be conducted. Our knowledge derives almost entirely from animal experiments, but it is impossible not to speculate on the possible implications in human breast cancer. It seems fairly certain that tumours excite a weak immune response, the breast being no exception, and that this response may be overwhelmed by a large volume of tumour cells. This would imply that it is desirable to excise as many tumour cells as possible, even if the excision were incomplete, so that the weak immune response had a task which was more within its capability. It has been shown experimentally that trauma, irradiation, starvation or intercurrent illness weaken the organism's resistance to tumour spread. This must make the thoughtful surgeon wonder how much damage his operations do to natural resistance and how much his radiotherapeutic colleague may be harming the patient. Chemical trauma by the administration of cytotoxic drugs must also enter this unsolved equation.

Crile[9] has advanced the view that local lymph nodes play an important part in providing an immune response to breast carcinoma. I find Crile's evidence unconvincing and the experimental work of Hammond and Rolley[10] indicates that the immune response is a function of the whole lympho-reticular system of the body and not merely of the regional lymph nodes. Here again we have a debated question which may well bear weightily on the matter of technique. Efforts to raise host resistance by such measures as B.C.G. vaccines, or the implanting of irradiated cells from the host's own tumour into his body are exciting possibilities which remain to be evaluated.

It is against this uncomfortable background of pathological fact and speculation that one has to weigh the advantages and disadvantages of the varying techniques which have been described. In this the ultimate result of a technique is of course the yardstick by which it is judged.

Evaluation of results

In comparing and contrasting the results of different techniques, the easiest yardstick to use is the duration of the patient's life after treatment. In Halsted's day a 3 year period free from recurrence was considered proof of cure. More recently a period of 5 years has been more cautiously adopted. But it is now widely recognised that it is necessary to have a 10 year follow-up before there can be any strong hope of cure. Even then the

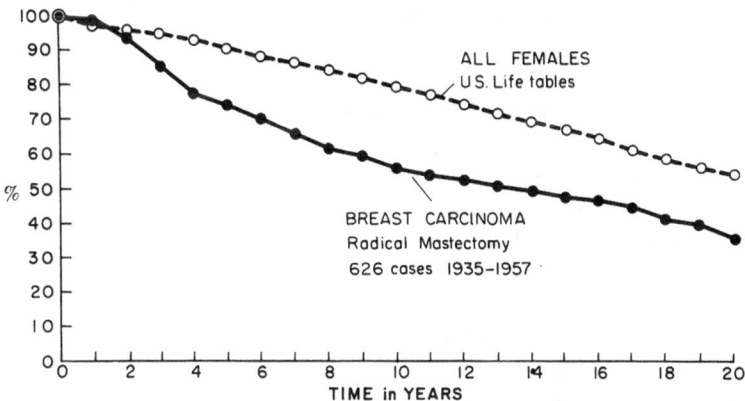

Figure 2.1 Dr Haagensen's survival curve for those with carcinoma of the breast treated by radical mastectomy, compared with survival of all women in New York State. (Reproduced from Haagensen[11], by kind permission of the author and W. B. Sanders Co.)

occasional patient will show recurrences for the first time long after the tenth anniversary of her operation. It seems reasonable however to adopt a 10-year period as the yardstick. Haagensen (Figure 2.1)[11] has shown that the life expectation of a group of breast cancer patients begins to run parallel with the mortality of the general population after the tenth post-operative year. This considerable interval clearly makes a final judgement on any technique a long-delayed affair.

There are difficulties even in judging the length of life. It is often impossible to be quite sure whether or not a patient died of her breast cancer or of some other disease. Surgeons have usually recorded their results as the crude death rate, all patients dying being counted as dead from the carcinoma. Those with more sophisticated mathematical minds have sometimes adjusted the death rate of a group by subtracting the natural death rate of groups of the same age, as quoted in such tables as the Registrar General publishes. This will of course improve the results and it is necessary to know whether an author has done this before judging his results.

As has been remarked, it is not only the length of life of a patient with breast carcinoma which counts. The quality of her life is also of great importance; and hitherto, perhaps owing to the difficulty of measuring quality, less attention has been paid to it. In considering the merits of one technique as contrasted with another, some attempt at least should be made to assess quality. Two easily measured standards are the state of the patient's arm on the operated side as regards swelling and movement; and the local recurrence rate. To survive for long periods with a large fungating ulcer, requiring daily dressing, may to some be a fate worse than death. Almost impossible to measure but also clearly of great importance to the quality of a patient's life is the psychological reaction to her treatment.

The appraisal of techniques

Because of the uncertainty which so surprisingly still exists as to the best method of treating the earlier or operable case of breast cancer, attempts have been made to judge the results by comparing series of cases treated by different methods. There are two principal ways in which this has been done, the retrospective comparison and the clinical trial.

RETROSPECTIVE COMPARISON

For this (as also with clinical trials) it is essential that the patients should have been sorted into approximately comparable groups by careful clinical staging, using identical criteria for staging. The results obtained by one technique in one centre can then be compared with the results of another technique in another centre. Perhaps the best example of this method is Haagensen's co-operative international study of results from 7 different centres, each using one technique, but employing an identical method of staging[12]. Criticism has been levelled at this method on 2 counts. The first is that there may be widely differing standards of clinical acumen and operative expertise between one centre and another. The second is that the genetic consti-tution and the environmental surroundings of a population in one country may make a significant difference to the results of treatment in a population at the opposite side of the world.

Other trials of a similar nature have come in for more severe criticism. Thus Anglem and Leber[13] have shown that the well-known papers of Crile, in which he has advocated sim-ple mastectomy and radiotherapy as the treatment of choice for breast cancer, show evidence of bias in case selection which favoured the simple operation. These authors have also criti-cised the papers of Rissanen[14] in that the size of tumour in the conservatively treated group was much smaller than in the radically treated group and thus favoured the result of the con-servative method which Rissanen was advocating.

It is clear that, in drawing any conclusion from retro-spective comparisons, the surgeon must be wary of the uncon-scious bias which is liable to trap enthusiastic authors.

CLINICAL TRIALS

At the present time the most widely used and most popular way of trying to evaluate techniques of treatment is the clinical trial. In this, patients are randomly selected for one of two methods of treatment at the same centre. Five such trials are currently being conducted on a large scale in the United Kingdom and many more in the United States, as also, no doubt, in other parts of the world. It will be some time before the 10-year results of these trials are available in sufficient quantities to have a sig-nificant meaning. Clinical trials are exceedingly difficult to conduct and many of the smaller ones which have been reported have run into serious criticism. Thus Anglem and Leber[13] have uncovered serious deficiencies, revealing unconscious bias in favour of the argument which an author was advocating. In the well-known clinical trial of Kaae and Johansen[15], which was designed to show that no difference in the 5-year result could be seen between the McWhirter method and extended radical mastectomy, Anglem and Leber[13] show that the 10 year survival was better for extended radical mastectomy even though this group contained a smaller percentage of Stage A cases, and they also point out that 25 of the 206 patients in the extended radical group did not in fact have this operation at all, though they were used in calculating the survival figures.

Once again it is obvious that the clinical trial is an exceedingly difficult weapon to use properly, but it does nevertheless seem that it will in the end produce convincing and reliable data.

To turn now to the actual details of technique, it is perhaps pertinent first to discuss the technique of biopsy which must so frequently be done before certainty of diagnosis is established.

Biopsy

It is clearly of importance to offer as little local disturbance as possible to a malignant tumour and to create as little local disfigurement as is consistent with one's objective if the lump should happily prove to be benign. For surgical biopsies curved incisions over the lump, which run parallel with the edge of areola, lie in the natural lines of Langer and they heal with a minimum of scarring—radial incisions are to be avoided. Biopsy of small malignant tumours must be by excision, but larger ones are less disturbed by cutting into them and removing a piece for the pathologist. Haemostasis in biopsy cavities must be meticulous and is best achieved with dissecting diathermy forceps, and the skin closed by a continuous suture. This will prevent oozing of blood or tissue fluid laden with malignant cells into the area of a larger operation which may necessarily follow. A further precaution against malignant contamination of a larger wound is of course to sew a swab, wrung out in antiseptic solution, over a biopsy incision as the first step after the re-towelling and change of gloves and instruments has been done.

Needle biopsy is a less traumatic alternative to surgical biopsy. Its disadvantage is that only a positive result is useful. When a needle biopsy fails to reveal malignancy, it is not possible to be sure that the needle has hit the right place. As one who has little experience of the method, I must concede that my dislike of needle biopsy may be prejudiced; it does have a place in those large inoperable tumours where pathological proof is required before a course of radiotherapy is to be the prime therapy.

Before considering the various techniques which have been proposed for the surgical treatment of breast cancer, a brief discussion on what is meant by the "operable case" is required.

Surgery and clinical staging

While there is much debate about what form surgery should take in the "operable" case, there is less controversy about those patients who should or should not be treated primarily by operation. It is for example generally conceded that the inflammatory carcinoma is not suitable for any operation beyond biopsy and that operation may speed the malignant process in these very rapidly growing cancers. It is also widely accepted that it is only patients in Stage 1 or 2 (A or B in the Columbia Staging) who are suitable for operation and that the later stages should receive radiotherapy only, or modification of the hormone balance or, in the most advanced stages, by chemotherapy, with surgery in a minor and ancillary role as a toilette for ulceration. There are however some who believe that the surgical removal of large tumour masses is worthwhile in terms of patient comfort even when there is clearly no hope of cure. Too rigid an application of the rules of clinical staging to surgery is to be avoided and one has to remember that clinical staging is in any event a highly inaccurate process.

It used to be thought that pregnancy and lactation were a contraindication to surgery. Carcinomata occurring at this time are not usually of the inflammatory type and these patients have as good a prospect of cure if their axillary lymph nodes are free as in the generality of cases. If the nodes are involved the prognosis becomes considerably more gloomy.

Tylectomy (lumpectomy)

Local excision of malignant tumours has been practised for hundreds of years, has been shown by itself to yield deplorable results and has only come again into consideration because of the advent, within the range of living memory, of effective radiotherapy. This latter has made a reappraisal of the situation both appropriate and necessary.

Tylectomy, as a serious proposition, seems to have begun in 1954 with the paper of Mustakollio, when he advocated a local or wedge excision followed by radiotherapy for tumours when they were localised and could be easily extirpated. Rissanen[14] has recently reported the continuation of this work, and contrasted tylectomy and radiotherapy with radical mastectomy. As already pointed out, the tylectomy group showed selection of the more favourable cases for the procedure; yet the 5- and 10-year survival rate was about equal and there was a 26% recurrence rate in the affected breast after tylectomy.

Atkins and his colleagues[16] at Guy's Hospital have been engaged in a trial of tylectomy with radiotherapy versus radical mastectomy with radiotherapy. They reported in 1972 that the results of tylectomy were significantly worse in those patients with clinically involved axillary nodes (both in regard to local and distant recurrence, and survival) than after radical mastectomy. There was also a higher incidence of local recurrence after tylectomy in patients with clinically uninvolved axillary nodes, but the distant recurrence rate and the survival in this Stage 1 group did not differ from that following radical mastectomy.

I have myself used tylectomy with radiotherapy for well defined indications. Where the patient is very old or seriously impaired in health from some other disease, where she refuses more rádical surgery, or where the growth is situated on the extreme inner edge of the breast disc, a wedge resection seems justified.

The greatly increased local recurrence rate, the finding by the Guy's group that distant metastasis is more frequent and survival time less in the Stage 2 case do not seem to me to justify tylectomy with radiotherapy as the usual and proper technique for the average early case, particularly when one remembers the 30–40% error which the clinician makes in his assessment of the invasion of or freedom from carcinoma of the axillary nodes.

Simple mastectomy

Simple mastectomy as a treatment for the earlier cases of breast cancer had virtually disappeared under the influence of Halsted until the work of McWhirter (stimulated by the example of Keynes at St. Bartholomew's Hospital) aroused interest in it as a combined procedure with radiotherapy. McWhirter first published his views in 1948 and provoked heated and even acrimonious discussion. He gained a considerable following and even now the place of simple mastectomy and radiotherapy remains unsettled until the late results of proper clinical trials are to hand. There has been considerable support for McWhirter's ideas. Brinkley and Haybittle[17] found no difference in 204 patients who entered their trial between simple and radical mastectomy, with radiotherapy to both groups. This trial was however small and the maximum time of follow up of 6 years was not only too short but also did not apply to all the patients, many of whom had been followed for a considerably shorter time.

Crile[9] is perhaps the best known advocate of simple mastectomy in the United States. He does not give additional radiotherapy to the majority of his clinical Stage 1 patients. Where axillary recurrence is found in these patients, local excision of the recurrent nodes is done, often with the addition of radiotherapy. Crile maintains that the results of simple mastectomy are superior to those of radical mastectomy and Chapter 5 of his book[9] marshals an impressive body of evidence to support his contentions. Reference has however already been made to the criticism which Anglem and Leber have made of Crile's statistics.

Notable among the evidence to show that simple mastectomy is not as good an operation as radical mastectomy is Haagensen's co-operative international study[12] wherein it was found that the 10-year survival rate for simple mastectomy with radiotherapy for Stage A cases was 40% as compared with the 60–70% 10-year survival in the more radically treated series.

Miller's[12] patients however received a dose of radiotherapy which would today be considered quite inadequate.

I myself am impressed by the frequency with which I see, as a second opinion, patients with axillary recurrences after simple mastectomy. Axillary recurrence after simple mastectomy and radiotherapy is a disaster which is scarcely ever seen after more radical procedures. It is very difficult to know what to do, or whether further radiotherapy is possible, especially if the axillary involvement has begun to cause lymphoedema of the arm.

Further clinical trials are proceeding both here, in the USA, and elsewhere as to the place of simple mastectomy. In the British trials, so far as they have gone, the survival time seems not to be much different from more radical procedures. Post-operative morbidity is greater for the radical operation but chest wall and axillary recurrence is greater for the simple procedures. It is to be hoped that when 10-year results are available, some effort will be made to estimate the quality as well as the quantity of survival.

Radical mastectomy

Since Halsted first advocated radical mastectomy in 1893 it has been the most widely practised of all the operative treatments for breast cancer. When Halsted first described it there was no radiotherapy and in cases which we should now deem inoperable he had no other choice. The virtue of the operation was that it gave excellent access to the axilla and there can be no doubt that Halsted's results were a great improvement on those of his contemporaries. The disadvantage of the operation in modern eyes is the added mutilation which is involved in removing the pectoralis major as well as the breast. Radical mastectomy probably remains the most widely practised operation throughout the world and is still the principal yardstick in clinical trials against which alternative operations are judged. Its most renowned advocate today is Haagensen[12] who in his co-operative international study has shown results which have never been equalled. He showed a 69% 10-year survival in 344 Stage A cases. Other authors have recently supported the Halsted mastectomy as the treatment of choice. Lee and Lambley[18] showed a 60% 10-year survival in their 200 Stage 1 cases and

Butcher[12] a 56% 10-year survival in 216 Stage A cases. There are, however, many who contend that simple mastectomy with radiotherapy produces equally good survival. Thus, Williams, Murley and Curwen[19] in a large but not very homogeneous series from St. Bartholomew's Hospital found little difference between the two operations in survival time. They found, as many others have done, that morbidity was lower after the simpler procedure but local recurrence less after the radical operation.

Conservative radical mastectomy

In speaking of conservative radical mastectomy, I must declare an interest. It is an operation, originally described by Patey and Dyson[20], which I have for many years practised and advocated. Readers must bear in mind Professor MacNeill Dixon's words: "There never yet was a philosopher, whatever they may have said, no, nor man of science, whose conclusions ran counter to the dearest wishes of his heart, who summed up against them, or condemned his hopes to death".

When Thackray and I began to find in 1948, as a result of our biopsy studies, that lymph nodes in the internal mammary chain were invaded in about 25% of "operable" cases, it seemed to us that radical mastectomy was not radical at all, in that it failed to ablate a subsidiary but nevertheless important primary lymph drainage system. We therefore adopted Patey's technique in the belief that it caused less mutilation than Halsted's operation while securing the admitted though limited advantages of the latter. The cardinal point in the technique is the preservation of the pectoralis major muscle, which can be sufficiently relaxed if the arm is raised to point towards the ceiling to permit excision of the pectoralis minor muscle and complete clearance of the axilla up to the first rib. The only point which needs more special care than in the classical technique is the preservation of the pectoral branch of the thoraco–acromial artery and the lateral pectoral nerve which runs with it: this ensures a blood and nerve supply to the pectoralis major without which its preservation is pointless. We also added biopsies of the internal mammary lymph nodes, not as a therapy but as a pathological reconnaisance, and this of course is no part of the

original technique. The only possible point in which this technique is inferior to Halsted's is that the interpectoral lymph
nodes of Rotter are not cleared cleanly because they lie in close
proximity to the pectoral artery and nerve. The lower part of
the pectoralis major is also partly paralysed because the medial
pectoral nerve runs through the pectoralis minor muscle and
must be sacrificed with that muscle.

The great advantage of the technique is cosmetic. It
involves no more mutilation than a simple mastectomy and
patients are not hollow below the clavicle. With some slight
attention to detail, conventional evening and swimming cloth-
ing can be worn after the operation. We have seen one recurrence in the pectoralis major in about 800 cases. Of the 159
Stage A cases who passed the 10th anniversary of their operation
100 (63%) were alive, and this compares well with other series
of Halsted operations except for that of Haagensen.

There have been various modifications of the conservative
radical mastectomy, all tending to be more conservative still
and perhaps deserving rather the title of extended simple
mastectomies. Thus Auchincloss[21] clears only the lateral axilla,
leaving the pectoralis minor intact. His contention is that
patients with pathological proven invasion of the apical axillary
nodes do badly after the full radical operation and it is therefore
not worth clearing the apex of the axilla: if the apical nodes are
clear, there is no point in removing them and if invaded it makes
no difference anyhow. Auchincloss has not yet had time to provide statistical evidence on the outcome of his modification.
Madden[22] has also used a somewhat similar technique in which
both pectoral muscles are preserved, but his paper provided no
statistical evidence of results.

Extended radical mastectomy

When Thackray and I first began to realise the implications of
invasion of the internal mammary lymph nodes, it did not
appear to us possible to excise the nodes in an "en bloc" operation. That this was not so was demonstrated conclusively by
Urban[23] who is the chief protagonist of the extended radical
operation. He has shown a 60% crude survival rate at 10 years
in 262 operable patients. The word "operable" must be pre-
sumed to refer to Stages 1 and 2 but Urban has not given his

results in a way in which the 2 earlier clinical stages can be separated. Nevertheless this represents an excellent result. Others have had a less favourable experience. Dahl Iversen and Tobiassen[24] fared no better with an extended radical technique than other surgeons using less extensive operations; but it is only fair to say that their operation was not the "en bloc" procedure used by Urban. Caceres[25] could not demonstrate any added value in the extended mastectomy which he performed. Donegan[26], in a very complete independent study of the results of Sugarbaker's extended mastectomy and my series of conservative mastectomies, found virtually no difference in the ultimate results.

It does not seem that extended radical mastectomies should be generally adopted. Except in skilful and well practised hands it would certainly carry a higher mortality and morbidity than less drastic procedures if it were done in small units which had no special interest in breast disease.

Conclusion

I have already referred to Sir Hedley Atkins' remark in 1953 that the method of treatment for operable breast cancers made a difference to the end result in only some 10% of cases. In a disease whose treatment has caused so much discussion and controversy, it seems that this is likely to be true. If any one method of treatment was greatly superior to all others, it must have been recognised long ago. One has only to recollect, for example, the introduction of penicillin to remember its instant acceptance as something far superior to anything which had gone before. Until we have settled the vexed question of what our present methods can do—until in fact we solve the biochemical question about malignant tumours which will enable us to substitute injections for operations and radiotherapy—it would seem a mistake for the surgeon who operates on few cases of breast cancer each year to abandon conventional teaching; he should use radical mastectomy with proper clearance of the axilla or one of its modifications.

This is not to denigrate the clinical trials at present proceeding. They are of the utmost importance but the difficulty of conducting them makes them suitable only for large institutions with access to large numbers of cases and backed by proper statistical expertise. It is not enough to enjoy the comfort of opinion without the discomfort of thought or the dedicated hard labour which a clinical trial involves. Too many surgeons have advocated one or other method of treatment without producing evidence which stands up to critical scrutiny. It seems then that, in our present state of uncertainty, the surgeon who has no specialised interest in the treatment of breast cancer should use the conservative radical mastectomy, supplementing it with radiotherapy if the histologist reports that the axillary lymph nodes are invaded.

I would end by a brief extract from Professor MacNeill Dixon's 1935 Gifford Lectures:

"If you find my conclusions unpalatable, you are not without resource. You have only to assure yourselves that I am totally mistaken, which may, indeed, very likely be the truth. And — who knows? — I may learn wisdom and come to think differently." I shall not come to think differently unless you produce convincing evidence that I am mistaken, and the evidence will have to include the quality as well as the quantity of survival.

REFERENCES

1. Dobson, J. (1972). Percival Pott. *Ann. Roy. Coll. Surg. Eng.*, **50**, 54
2. Fisher, B. and Fisher, E. R. (1967). Barrier function of lymph node to tumor cells and erythrocytes. *Cancer*, **20**, 1907
3. Galasko, C. S. B. (1969). The detection of skeletal metastases from mammary cancer by gamma camera scintigraphy. *Brit. J. Surg.*, **56**, 757
4. Roberts, S. S., Hangesh, J. W., McGrath, R. G., Valaitis, J., McGrew, E. and Cole, W. H. (1967). Prognostic significance of cancer cells in the circulating blood: a ten year evaluation. *Amer. J. Surg.*, **113**, 757
5. Handley, R. S. (1972). Observations and thoughts on cancer of the breast. *Proc. Roy. Soc. Med.*, **65**, 437
6. Qualheim, R. E. and Gall, E. A. (1957). Breast carcinoma with multiple sites of origin. *Cancer*, **10**, 460
7. Muir, R. (1941). Evolution of carcinoma of mamma. *J. Path. Bact.*, **52**, 155
8. Gallager, H. S. and Martin, J. E. (1969). Early phases in the development of breast cancer. *Cancer*, **24**, 1170
9. Crile, G., Jr. (1967). *A Biological Consideration of Treatment of Breast Cancer*. Springfield, Illinois: Charles C. Thomas
10. Hammond, W. G. and Rolley, R. T. (1970). Retained regional lymph nodes: effect upon metastases and recurrence after tumor removal. *Cancer*, **25**, 368
11. Haagensen, C. D. (1971). *Diseases of the Breast*. Philadelphia: W. B. Sanders Co.

12. Haagensen, C. D. *et al.* (1969). Treatment of early mammary carcinoma: a cooperative international study. *Ann. Surg.*, **170**, 875

13. Anglem, T. J. and Leber, R. E. (1972). The dubious case for conservative operation in operable cancer of the breast. *Ann. Surg.*, **176**, 625

14. Rissanen, P. M. (1969). A comparison of conservative and radical surgery combined with radiotherapy in the treatment of Stage 1 carcinoma of the breast. *Brit. J. Radiol.*, **42**, 423

15. Kaae, S. and Johansen, H. (1969). Simple mastectomy plus post-operative irradiation by the method of McWhirter for mammary carcinoma. *Ann. Surg.*, **170**, 895

16. Atkins, Sir H. *et al.* (1972). Treatment of early breast cancer: a report after ten years of a clinical trial. *Brit. Med. J.*, **ii**, 423

17. Brinkley, D. and Haybittle, J. L. (1966). Treatment of Stage 11 carcinoma of the female breast. *Lancet*, **ii**, 291

18. Lee, R. O. and Lambley, D. G. (1971). Radical mastectomy in the treatment of breast cancer. A follow-up study over ten and fifteen years. *Brit. J. Surg.*, **58**, 137

19. Williams, I. G., Murley, R. S. and Curwen, M. P. (1953). Carcinoma of the female breast: conservative and radical surgery. *Brit. Med. J.*, **ii**, 787

20. Patey, D. H. and Dyson, W. H. (1948). The prognosis of carcinoma of the breast in relation to the type of operation performed. *Brit. J. Cancer*, **2**, 7

21. Auchincloss, H. (1963). Significance of location and number of axillary metastases in carcinoma of the breast: a justification for a conservative operation. *Ann. Surg.*, **158**, 37

22. Madden, J. L. (1965). Modified radical mastectomy. *Surg. Gynae. and Obst.*, **121**, 1221

23. Urban, J. A. and Castro, E. B. (1971). Selecting variations in extent of surgical procedure for breast cancer. *Cancer*, **28**, 1615

24. Dahl Iversen, E. and Tobiassen, T. (1963). Radical mastectomy with parasternal and supraclavicular dissection for mammary carcinoma. *Ann. Surg.*, **157**, 170

25. Caceres, E. (1967). An evaluation of radical mastectomy and extended radical mastectomy for cancer of the breast. *Surg. Gynae. Obst.*, **125**, 337

26. Donegan, W. L. (1972). Mastectomy in the primary management of invasive mammary carcinoma. *Advances in Surgery* (J. D. Hardy, editor). Year Book Publishers Inc. Chicago

3

Radiotherapy

M. D. Snelling

It is now universally accepted that the treatment of any individual patient suffering from carcinoma of the breast, as from any other form of malignant disease, requires the collaboration and repeated consultation of specialists of many disciplines.

Surgeons, radiotherapists, chemotherapists, endocrinologists and immunologists are all involved, as are also many of their clinical colleagues, as well as pathologists, radiologists and biochemists, experts in nuclear medicine, thermography, ultrasound and many others.

Each case requires repeated individual assessment if the many different possibilities of therapy are to be used to the best advantage.

The basic philosophy of radiotherapy is similar to that of surgery — complete elimination of primary growth and regional lymphatic metastases by physical means — in surgery by ablation and in radiotherapy by the death of all malignant cells as a result of physical changes, mostly in the nucleus, produced by ionising radiation. Once the disease is widespread and cure no longer possible, palliative therapy by incomplete destruction of tumour masses is of value and will be considered in a separate section.

"Cure" of malignant disease is difficult to define since even where the disease is apparently completely eradicated on the chest wall and in the regional glandular areas, distant metastases or local recurrence may appear after many years and it is recognised that in carcinoma of the breast survival rates are very similar following all the commonly used forms of management of the disease. Until, however, more is known of the mechanisms of immunology and until the results of scientific trials comparing localised treatment and regional therapy are available, it is accepted by many radiotherapists that radical therapy to primary or to the whole region comprising primary tumour and glands, is of great value and that whenever such treatment is given it should be in a dosage and time found by experience to cause complete destruction of all carcinoma cells in the volume to which it is delivered. Inadequate treatment cannot destroy the disease and while short term palliation is achieved, it is followed by recurrence.

Theory of radiotherapy

The effect of ionising radiation on living cells was noted very soon after X-rays had been discovered by Röentgen and γ rays by Madame Curie at the end of the last century. This effect is greatest on dividing cells and therefore in normal tissue on the marrow and seminal tubules where new cells are produced continuously at a high rate. The skin and mucous membrane, where the basal cells divide continuously to replace shed epithelium, are more sensitive to irradiation than are the cells of muscle and connective tissues where mitosis is infrequent or absent — this accounts for the well-known "skin reaction".

Radiotherapy involves the administration of a prescribed quantity of ionising energy to a block of tissue containing malignant and normal cells and, where the difference in radiosensitivity is sufficient, the tumour cells are destroyed and the normal tissues, although scarred, are so only to a tolerable extent.

The radiosensitivity of different tumours varies widely and depends not only on the rate of mitosis but also very importantly upon the oxygenation of the cells. An anaplastic carcinoma is far more sensitive than is a more slowly growing adenocarcinoma, while the highly vascular "inflammatory" carcinoma will respond more quickly and completely than will the comparatively avascular scirrhous carcinoma.

In general, however, carcinoma of the breast is relatively avascular and slowly growing, and therefore a high dose of irradiation is required. Various devices, however, are available by which sensitivity of the tumour relative to the tolerance of the tumour bed is increased.

The dose or quantity of radiation delivered is limited by the volume of the tissue irradiated — where this is too large, as when the whole breast is infiltrated by tumour—complete destruction by irradiation may be impossible, although an inoperable tumour may be made operable by the treatment. The tolerance of the patient and the local tolerance of the normal tissues may, however, be increased by increasing the total duration of the treatment and by splitting the total dose into a number of fractions. A high dose is therefore usually delivered in fractions which vary from daily to weekly, while the total duration of the treatment runs from three to eight weeks. This wide variation shows our present uncertainty as to how to achieve a balance between radiation injury and repair in normal and neoplastic tissues, and much research is currently being done on this subject by radiotherapists and radiobiologists.

In each episode of irradiation the more sensitive oxygenated tumour cells receive lethal injury while the anoxic cells survive. In the interval between the treatments some recovery of surviving cells occurs, while fresh vascularisation following the death and removal of the sensitive oxygenated cells results in improved oxygenation of the previously anoxic radio-resistant cells in the centre of the tumour, which then become more sensitive to subsequent treatments.

The possibilities of complete destruction of these avascular tumours provided by different regimes of total dose, overall duration of treatment and number, spacing and dosage of individual treatments is of intense interest to both clinical radiotherapists and radiobiologists.

In avascular tumours where it appears impossible to deliver the necessary dose, attempts have been made to increase the sensitivity of the tumour by placing the patient before and during treatment in a plastic chamber where she breathes oxygen with a suitable addition of carbon dioxide at a pressure of 3 atmospheres. The value of this method of sensitisation is being currently assessed by the Medical Research Council in Britain.

In recent years there has been increasing interest in the use of chemotherapy in the treatment of carcinoma of the.breast. It is already apparent that pulsed chemotherapy with many agents used synchronously or consecutively is sometimes of great value in recurrent local and in disseminated disease and it may later prove to be of value also in the earlier stages of the disease (see Chapter 1).

When prescribing the treatment of any patient a radiotherapist must consider the purpose of the treatment — curative or palliative — the volume to be irradiated, the total quantity of ionising energy to be delivered, the total time and fractionation to be employed. He must also decide the physical qualities of the rays he wishes to use and the various technical problems concerned with the accurate localisation of the treatment.

Modalities of radiotherapy

Excluding neutron therapy which is being investigated and which may be found to be of value in the treatment of hypoxic cells, the effects of all available ionising radiations are considered identical and proportional to the energy absorbed in the irradiated tissues. The difference in pattern of ionisation and absorption produced by different beams varies with different energies and makes the radiation physicist an essential member of the team.

The choice of beam depends essentially upon the dimensions, site, and volume to be irradiated — and upon the dimensions of the patient. In most radiotherapy centres γ rays from units containing radiocobalt sources — rather more penetrating than the γ rays of radium — and equivalent approximately to X-rays produced at a voltage of about two million volts are used. This beam has a penetrating power adequate for all but the largest breasts and has the advantage of producing less skin reaction than do conventional 250 kV X-rays — a full effect on infiltrated skin can, however, be produced if desired. Highly filtered 250 kV X-rays have only sufficient penetrating power to treat small breasts and even then the skin reaction often limits the dosage to that below the dose necessary to destroy the tumour. Where a large patient has an extensive tumour filling one breast even ^{60}Co γ rays cannot give adequate irradiation and more penetrating X-rays from a linear accelerator with energies of several million volts are necessary — there are, however, technical difficulties in producing the exact effect desired on the skin overlying the tumour.

Adequate treatment of carcinoma of the breast requires a wide variation in techniques and equipment and is made difficult by the variations not only in the tumour but also in the size and shape of different patients—individualisation and strict accuracy are essential but richly repay the care and time of radiotherapist and radiographer.

Treatment by combination of surgery and radiotherapy

While the philosophy of management will continue to vary greatly in different centres—and with different individuals—until the results of the current controlled trials of localised and regional therapy are known, the object of any combination of surgery and radiotherapy must be the complete removal or destruction of the disease in the selected areas of primary site and glands. Where either discipline is concerned, to give less than adequate therapy not only leaves residual disease, but also reduces the local resistance of the tumour bed to the malignant process.

Where radiotherapy is used, the selected area which may consist of the whole region, the chest wall alone, or individual glandular areas, should therefore receive a total dose shown by experience to be likely to destroy all neoplastic disease at that site. Since such treatment always involves a high dose of radiation, it is inevitably followed by fibrosis and by changes in irradiated blood vessels which lead to a degree of ischaemia of the skin and connective tissues. The inevitable irradiation of the lung is reduced to the minimum by the use of tangential, glancing irradiation of the chest wall, but fibrosis and sometimes fracture of the ribs is common and some degree of underlying fibrosis of the lung may occur. Where residual disease remains after radical surgery, the radiosensitivity of the remaining cancer cells is decreased by the impairment of the blood supply and it appears sometimes that the diminished resistance of the irradiated normal skin to carcinomatous invasion favours the growth of residual cells here as compared with the adjoining unirradiated skin.

After attempted clearance of the axilla by surgery, residual glands in an area of post-surgical fibrosis and impaired blood supply are also resistant to radiation and are unlikely to be destroyed by a dose of radiation tolerated by the damaged normal tissues.

The addition of full radiotherapy to a site of failed radical surgery is, therefore, unlikely to succeed as a method of salvage; while the combined post-surgery and post-irradiation changes lead to troublesome sequelae and possibly even favour later growth of temporarily quiescent carcinoma cells. In spite of these difficulties combination of surgery and radiotherapy has often resulted in at least regional cure of disease which has progressed beyond that removed adequately by surgery alone.

In order, however, to provide some individual patient with the optimum treatment at present available, her management should be planned initially by surgeon and radiotherapist together, after full preliminary investigations have been performed. The presence of bilateral disease and distal spread must be investigated and an accurate assessment made of site and extent of the tumour, presence and extent of any glandular metastases, and also a clinical assessment of the malignancy of the tumour.

Mammography is being increasingly useful and may be supplemented by ultrasound studies and by thermography. Aspiration cytology is also useful at this stage to confirm the malignancy of the primary tumour, or the presence of gland involvement (see Chapter 1).

A decision can then be made by surgeon and radiotherapist together upon the part to be played by each in the treatment of the patient. Where for practical reasons such consultations are not always possible, the policies to be followed and the principles relating management and techniques to the clinical findings must have been agreed and clearly defined. Since therapy by any means must be exactly prescribed and carried out, and prescriptions vary widely under different clinical conditions, a system which has operated over many years whereby a patient on whom a mastectomy has been performed for an undiscussed carcinoma is given "blanket" radical radiotherapy to wound and glands by a radiotherapist, should be totally condemned.

Post-operative radiotherapy in each case should be based on the likelihood of residual disease at different sites, and on the desirability of avoiding the irradiation of areas where the tumour has been completely removed.

Combinations of surgery and radiotherapy at present in use are the following:

1. Variations of radical mastectomy plus irradiation
2. Simple mastectomy plus irradiation
3. Local excision plus irradiation (this and treatment by irradiation alone are described later)
4. Pre-operative irradiation
5. Treatment of bilateral carcinoma
6. Radiotherapy for recurrent disease

1. Radical surgery and irradiation
The surgeon has removed the primary tumour and glands together with a margin, which has been decided after careful pre-operative assessment of the disease on the chest wall and in the axilla. After such surgery it is the author's practice to leave unirradiated the chest wall and lower axilla where recurrence after adequate surgery is rare, and where considerable morbidity may follow combined treatments. In cases where the lower axillary glands were involved the apical axillary and the sub- and supraclavicular glands are irradiated. Unless the internal mammary glands have been biopsied and found negative, they are included in the treatment, a dose of 5500 rad being given to the axillary nodes, and 5000 rad to the other glands during the course of 5 weeks, using γ rays from a ^{60}Co unit.

Where, owing to misjudgement, it appears at the operation that recurrence in the chest wall is likely, either because of the extent of the tumour or because of its malignancy, the chest wall is irradiated by tangential fields to a dosage of 5000 rad in $4\frac{1}{2}$ weeks — the skin is included in the treatment so that there is no sparing of the superficial layers and a desquamating skin reaction develops. Where the tumour was situated medially in the breast the internal mammary glands are included in the tangential irradiation. Where the tumour was lateral, it is treated by a separate direct anterior field continuous with the field covering supraclavicular region and anterior axilla. In some centres the chest wall and all the regional glands are irradiated in one block with a linear accelerator using X-rays produced at energies of several million volts.

2. Simple mastectomy followed by irradiation
Treatment techniques are similar to those already described, the volume to be treated being decided individually in each

case after consideration of the clinical findings and operative procedure. Where the full thickness of the skin covers the ribs over the whole of the area to be treated, a higher dose should be given and is well tolerated — for instance 5500 rad in 5 weeks, again without sparing the skin.

3. Local excision and treatment by radiotherapy alone are discussed in a separate section.

4. Pre-operative irradiation
Where a carcinoma of the breast is of obviously high malignancy but is apparently limited to the breast or to the lower axillary nodes, high dose regional radiotherapy should be followed by a planned simple mastectomy four or 6 weeks after the completion of treatment.

While the prognosis in such cases is always bad, occasional salvage is achieved. It is the author's practice to give a very high dose to the breast — 6500 or even 7500 rad in 6 or 7 weeks — using ^{60}Co teletherapy. Providing there is no evidence of distant spread, surgery is performed as soon as the reaction has subsided. Delayed post-irradiation fibrosis makes surgery more difficult and healing may be prolonged. More extensive surgery to breast or axilla is rarely advisable; sequelae are then common. Should the disease after irradiation remain too extensive for simple mastectomy, surgery should be avoided and further palliative radiotherapy considered.

Pre-operative irradiation may also be of value in the management of peripheral or large tumours of lower grade malignancy, providing that the glandular involvement is limited to the lower axilla.

5. Bilateral breast disease
In general the prognosis in such cases contra-indicates both radical surgery and high dose radiotherapy — irradiation to an adequate dosage of both breasts and all glandular areas would not be tolerated. The clinical condition having been fully assessed, surgeon and radiotherapist decide on the combination of treatment most likely to provide local and glandular control of the disease. In these cases simple mastectomy and localised irradiation of the glands are usually combined with hormone therapy. Chemotherapy is at present rarely used in the absence

of widespread disease, but recent developments in pulsed chemotherapy using many agents suggest that it may soon form an important part of the early management of extensive but still localised disease.

6. *Use of radiotherapy in the treatment of recurrent disease on the chest wall or in glandular areas*

(a) Local recurrence. Until the presence of metastases has been proved, local therapy is used, the dosimetry depending upon an estimation of both the obviously and the potentially involved areas. A wide margin is usually included. Dosage and technique depend upon the area and depth of the volume to be treated and upon any scarring of the tumour bed caused by previous surgery or irradiation. Treatment by superficial and deep X-rays, short distance ^{60}Co or ^{137}Cs teletherapy and electron beam therapy, all have their place, as does the traditional radium applicator — the radium, however, being now, for reasons of radioprotection, replaced by sources of ^{137}Cs or ^{192}Ir or, when remote loading equipment is available, by powerful sources of ^{60}Co. Radiotherapy is usually associated with the institution of hormonal control of the disease. While a second treatment if confined to a small area is sometimes useful, a third irradiation of any area should never be given — success is virtually impossible and post-irradiation sequelae almost certain. Local or parenteral chemotherapy should then be considered.

(b) Recurrence in previously irradiated glands in apex of axilla, supraclavicular region or thoracic inlet. Massive recurrence in these areas may cause pressure symptoms and should no relief follow hormone therapy, a further course of localised irradiation may be useful. Adequate penetration and sparing of the previously irradiated skin are both important and treatment should be with supervoltage X-rays from a linear accelerator, or failing this, γ rays from a ^{60}Co unit. Volume and dosage are limited by the effects of previous treatment and especially by the danger of producing a brachial plexus neuritis. Again, recent developments in chemotherapy promise alternative useful treatment.

The use of radiotherapy in the treatment of metastatic carcinoma is discussed in a later section.

Treatment of carcinoma of the breast by radiotherapy alone

While the use of radiotherapy alone has long been accepted in the treatment of advanced disease and of tumours of very high malignancy, there has recently been a revival of interest in the treatment of T_1 and T_2 tumours either by a combination of local excision followed by radical radiotherapy, or by radiotherapy alone.

This interest is especially great in France where at the Fondation Curie the work of Baclesse has been continued by Calle and Bataini, while Gros at Strasbourg directs a University Centre largely orientated to the diagnosis and treatment of breast disease. At a Symposium on the "non-mutilating" treatment of carcinoma of the breast held at Strasbourg in 1972, under the auspices of the European Association of Radiology, surgeons and radiotherapists from many hospitals and University centres in Europe and from the United States discussed the indications, techniques and results of this form of management of the disease. In recent years this has been made more effective by the many technological advances in equipment which have made possible a greatly increased dosage to the tumour than was possible by earlier "orthovoltage" (200–240 kV X-rays) techniques.

Since carcinoma of the breast is often a slow growing differentiated tumour in a poorly vascularised tumour bed, it is usually relatively radio resistant and a high tumour dose is essential. Although when treatment was restricted to deep X-rays the tumour dose was limited by the reaction of the overlying skin, it was demonstrated by Baclesse at the Fondation Curie in the Twenties, Thirties and Forties that the tumour dose could be raised by fractionating the treatment over a long period — patients attended five or six times each week for 3 months or more. Although the immediate results of such treatment were improved, the tolerance of the skin and tumour bed, as compared with that of the tumour, was very impressive. Late results were disappointing owing partly to the very advanced stage of the tumours referred for this type of treatment, and also owing to late sequelae, such as oedema, fibrosis and even necrosis resulting from the heavy irradiation of skin and tumour bed.

With the introduction of the ^{60}Co units and telecurietherapy the advantages of increased penetration and skin sparing made possible a rise in the tumour dose and a shortening in the total duration of the treatment, which resulted in an enhanced effect in the tumour. A tumour dose of 5000–6000 rad can now be given to the whole region including breast, chest wall, axillae, infra- and supraclavicular and internal mammary glands in a period of 5 or 6 weeks, the skin reaction exceeding an erythema only where this is deliberately produced because of infiltration of the skins. This is done by covering the area in the treatment.

While a dose of approximately 5500 rad in $5\frac{1}{2}$ weeks is adequate to destroy small foci of tumour, a higher dose has been found necessary where there are solid masses of tumour inevitably containing areas of poor vascularity and hypoxic cells. Because of this, an adequate local excision should be performed in T_1 or early T_2 cases before the irradiation, while in more extensive tumours where this is impossible, an additional 2500 to 3000 rad is delivered to the tumour after the completion of the regional irradiation. A tumour which, although small, is clinically of high malignancy and therefore unsuitable for primary local excision is similarly treated — in these cases the diagnosis is confirmed by drill biopsy after the administration of a dosage of 1500 rad. The method used for the administration of the final 2500–3000 rad depends upon the site of the tumour and the dosimetry required.

Where the skin is infiltrated and must receive the full dose an electron beam may be used, which penetrates to a depth determined by the energy used: where this is not available irradiation may be given by a small ^{60}Co or ^{137}Cs source positioned 10–20 cm from the skin — the fall off is then rapid because of the inverse square law. Where there is no apparent infiltration of the skin and the 5500-rad skin dose already received is considered to be sufficient, the underlying residual tumour mass is implanted with radioactive ^{192}Ir wire.

TREATMENT OF LYMPHATIC NODES

Axillary, infraclavicular, supraclavicular and internal mammary nodes all receive a dosage of 5500 rad in the initial regional irradiation. While this dosage may often be sufficient to destroy small masses of tumour a higher dosage would again be required for massive glandular involvement, but this may not always be possible because of the danger of late sequelae from irradiation of the normal tissues. While the dosage to localised masses in lower or middle axilla may be increased by an additional 1000 to 2000 rad, such treatment should be by small fields, and further irradiation of the brachial plexus in the apex of the axilla, or even more importantly in the neck, should be avoided because of the real danger of brachial neuritis and paralysis. Heavy irradiation of a mass of fixed glands filling the axilla is similarly contra-indicated by the possible production of fibrosis with oedema of the arm often made worse in such an advanced case with recurrence of the active growth.

While the results of these treatments will completely destroy the neoplasm in a large proportion of suitable cases, they should, because of the possible sequelae, be limited to those patients in whom this result may reasonably be expected. Where the cases are well chosen the results compare with those claimed by surgery and have the great psychological advantage of retaining a breast with little or no obvious scarring.

CHOICE OF CASE FOR "CONSERVATIVE TREATMENT"

It must be emphasised again that the object of the treatment is complete eradication of the disease in the breast and glandular areas. Where there are already distant metastases, or where only palliation of locally incurable disease is desired, simpler or less time-consuming palliative techniques should be used.

Treatment by local excision followed by radiotherapy

The indications for this treatment were discussed at the Strasbourg Symposium where it was agreed that it should be reserved for T_1 and early T_2 (under 3 cm) tumours without definite clinical evidence of axillary involvement (N_0 or N_{1A}). Calle (Fondation Curie) suggests absolute contra-indications as follows:

Bilateral disease
Tumours larger than 3 cm diameter
Multifocal disease
T_3 tumours

N_{1B} or more extensive glandular involvement

High malignancy

Papillon (Lyon) agrees on the importance of strict selection. He considers skin fixation to be a contra-indication and emphasises the importance of proving the absence of axillary gland involvement—if necessary by exploration. Adequate irradiation of a very large breast is impossible. Calle, Papillon and others have emphasised the importance of an adequate removal of the tumour, also the importance of previous mammography in the estimation of the size and extent of the tumour to be removed. Several authors maintain that the tumour should be at least 3 cm from the nipple. The author does not at present include $T_1 N_0$ or $T_1 N_{1B}$ cases without evidence of high malignancy where the tumour is in the lateral half of the breast and where the patient will accept mastectomy. These might be included when detailed results of the treatment are available.

Treatment of more advanced cases

While high dosage irradiation of extensive fixed or fungating tumour may prove a highly effective method of tumour control in inoperable disease, a very high dosage is necessary and care must be taken to weigh the advantages of the treatment against the possible late complications especially a possible brachial neuritis, oedema of the arm or necrosis of skin or bones. Such sequelae are, however, rare compared with the benefit which may follow carefully planned therapy, even where complete eradication of the disease is impossible.

High dosage is again essential: Calle describes the technique used at the Fondation Curie as follows (Personal communication):

Regional treatment to breast and lower axillary glands to a dosage of 6000 rad if given by ^{60}Co teletherapy. The remainder of the axilla, the infra- and supraclavicular glands and the internal mammary glands receive 5000 rad.

If the response is inadequate and surgery is possible, a mastectomy is performed after an interval of 8–12 weeks, but if it is satisfactory the volume treated is reduced and treatment continued to a total dose of 8000–8500 rad to the primary and to 6000, 7000 or even 7500 rad to the lower axilla.

The final part of the treatment is usually given by electron beam therapy.

Other techniques for the treatment of advanced cases in the United Kingdom have been described by Strickland (Mount Vernon Hospital) who gives a regional treatment with X-rays from a linear accelerator and by Sambrook (Swansea) who increases the tolerance of the normal tissues to a high dosage by a "split dose" technique in which an interval of a few weeks is given between the two halves of the treatment in order to allow some recovery of the irradiated normal tissues.

Results of treatment

The long term results await publication but it was reported by many delegates at the Strasbourg Symposium that the disease could be controlled locally in the majority of early cases, and that the majority of these controlled cases retained their breast. Calle (personal communication and in press) reports that of almost 300 $T_{1,2,3}$ cases with $N_{0,1A,1B}$ glands treated at the Fondation Curie between 1960 and 1966 approximately three-quarters were alive and two-thirds of the total showed no evidence of disease 5 years after the treatment. Of the last group two-thirds had retained the breast. Of 75 earlier cases ($T_{1,2}$ and $N_{0,1A}$) where the criteria described were strictly observed, 4 out of every 5 cases were alive and without evidence of disease, while 4 out of every 5 of these retained their breast.

He emphasises that salvage surgery is possible for local residual disease in breast and axilla, but also states that it is often difficult to diagnose active residual disease clinically, or by mammography, and that negative histology has been found after mastectomy on a number of occasions.

Calle states the cause of failure in two-thirds of the cases to have been distant metastases without evidence of residual disease at the primary site or in the glands. Complications were rare and the aesthetic result on which great importance is placed was good in 54 out of 116 cases and acceptable in 47 of the remaining cases.

Spitalier of Marseilles reported at Strasbourg a series of 185 strictly selected "operable" cases treated between 1961 and 1970 by local excision followed by 8000 rads external irradiation from a ^{137}Cs unit. In this group there were 15 failures

— 3 with contralateral carcinoma and 12 with metastases.

At The Middlesex Hospital a technique for the treatment of disease in the medial part of the breast has been developed similar in dosage to that used at the Fondation Curie. Similar results are being achieved. It is, however, our practice at The Middlesex when treating T_2 or T_3 cases of high malignancy always to follow regional irradiation, of 7000 or 8000 rad, by a mastectomy whenever possible without delay, since we believe that these rapidly growing tumours always recur.

Palliative therapy

Because of the long natural history of carcinoma of the breast patients suffering from this disease may live for many months and often years after the appearance of the first metastasis has indicated the inevitable fatal outcome. With adequate palliative treatment, which includes surgery, radiotherapy, hormone therapy and chemotherapy, many patients continue with an increasingly restricted but normal and satisfying life at home and in the community for a large proportion of this period of survival before the onset of a short final stage of complete incapacity.

Because of its importance in the relief of pain, dyspnoea and other symptoms of widespread disease, the treatment of metastatic carcinoma of the breast occupies much of the time of the radiotherapist, his team, his beds and his equipment.

Combination of radiotherapy with other disciplines
While hormone therapy is usually instituted after the proven appearance of the first metastasis with a view to controlling the disease as a whole, radiotherapy, combined sometimes with surgery, is used for the rapid control of symptoms caused by individual localised metastases. Its most important place is in the relief of pain and maintenance of mobility by the treatment of skeletal deposits, in the treatment of intrathoracic and intra-abdominal disease and in the control of cerebral and choroidal deposits, but local irradiation is of value also in shrinking metastases causing pressure symptoms in any part of the body. Its place in the treatment of recurrent local or glandular disease is described elsewhere.

Skeletal deposits
The management of skeletal disease is by a combination of hormone therapy and localised irradiation.

Local irradiation to a dosage of 2000 to 3000 rad over a period of 1–2 weeks is remarkably effective in reducing pain and producing sclerosis in osteolytic deposits. Where hospitalisation is impossible and the patient's general condition permits the inevitable reaction, a single treatment of 1000 rad to a localised area is equally effective. Such treatments will produce within a few days considerable relief of pain which relief increases steadily over 5 or 6 weeks, by which time the final effect is achieved — radiological evidence of sclerosis appears, however, only some weeks later. Retreatment of a skeletal metastasis is very rarely needed and it is interesting that such a small dose — compared with that needed for adequate therapy to the primary disease — should be so effective.

While treatment with 250 kV X-rays is effective, it has the disadvantage of low penetration and of producing a skin reaction in a decubitus patient. For this reason irradiation to the same dosage with a cobalt, or failing that, a caesium unit is to be preferred.

Any bone deposit causing pain may be irradiated and it is advisable also to irradiate prophylactically osteolytic disease in weight bearing bones where experience has shown collapse or fracture to be likely — such bones include vertebrae, the pelvis, sacro-iliac joints, acetabulum and the femur.

Irradiation of spinal metastases
While care must be taken to avoid radiation injury to the spinal cord, its tolerance which depends upon anatomical level, extent, and total duration of treatment, is usually above the dose necessary for adequate irradiation of the metastases. Irradiation of a large part of the spine produces marrow depression, but this is rarely important and may be corrected without difficulty by transfusion and steroids etc. An exception may occur where widespread small deposits are associated with leucoerythroblastic anaemia. Here pain is rarely a problem and treatment can only be with steroids, sometimes associated with chemotherapy. In many patients the whole length of the spine is irradiated thus enabling the patient to continue a restricted but

independent life. Where severe deformity has followed collapse a lumbar support is often of value, but a full length support for the thoracic spine is rarely tolerated by the patient.

Paraplegia
Where disease in the posterior part of the vertebral body or in the pedicles threatens paraplegia from pressure on the spinal cord, irradiation should not be instituted but the advice of the neurosurgeons should be called for immediately. Following successful surgical decompression local irradiation is indicated for residual disease in the spinal canal and vertebral body. Where a lower motor neurone weakness or parasthesia is due to pressure on the cauda equina, immediate decompression is not of prime importance and irradiation of the lumbar region is frequently followed by eventual recovery.

Pathological fracture of femur and humerus
Where there is a fracture of the shaft or neck of the femur, immobilisation of the patient is reduced to a few days by the insertion of a suitable internal support. Where the whole head and neck are infiltrated by neoplasm they are removed and replaced by a prosthesis — the choice of procedure depending upon the extent of the disease and the necessity for the presence of uninvolved bone. The surgery should be followed by irradiation. Similar management reduces the period of incapacity due to extensive disease or pathological fracture of the humerus.

Intrathoracic disease
Metastatic disease may occur in the pleural cavity, parenchyma of the lungs or mediastinum. Management is by a combination of hormone therapy, chemotherapy and radiotherapy, the first two being of greater importance than the last, except where glandular masses or infiltration are compressing trachea or bronchi, or rarely, oesophagus.

Pleural disease
Removal of the fluid is followed by local chemotherapy which may be repeated. Where the response is inadequate the intrapleural injection of 100 millicuries of colloidal radioactive gold has proved of value, but because of the necessary measures for

radioprotection is a more complicated procedure and to be used only when the simpler chemotherapeutic treatment has failed. It is now rarely used.

Where pleural infiltration is continuous with recurrent disease on the chest wall, external irradiation may relieve pain but is rarely followed by prolonged control.

Parenchymal disease in the lung is not controlled by irradiation and a combination of hormone therapy and chemotherapy is to be preferred.

Mediastinal involvement and lymphangitis carcinomatosa at the hilum causes distressing cough and dyspnoea. However, therapy is rarely effective but pulsed chemotherapy using a combination of agents combined with the administration of steroids sometimes gives temporary relief.

Where massive disease causes pressure symptoms, local irradiation in a dosage of 2500 or 3000 rad in 10–20 days may give considerable relief and is worth trying. Recurrent laryngeal nerve palsy rarely recovers following any treatment.

Cerebral metastases

The distressing symptoms of these metastases, which are always multiple, may incapacitate a patient many weeks or even months before her death but can in most cases be permanently relieved by adequate therapy. Such treatment prolongs the patient's active life without increasing the terminal bedridden phase, and by its relief of distressing symptoms, may prove of inestimable benefit to patient and relatives.

Management is by steroids combined with radiotherapy. Following the administration of dexamethasone 2 mg four times a day, a dose of 3000 rad is given to the whole of the cerebrum, including the posterior fossa. In those cases where clinical signs and brain scan indicate an apparently large deposit, this may receive 3500 rad and the remainder of the brain 2500. The duration of the treatment is determined by the patient's reaction — headache, papilloedema and level of consciousness, and usually lasts 3 or 4 weeks.

The inevitable irradiation of all hair follicles produces complete baldness, of which the patient must be warned. Shaving of the scalp before the treatment reduces the superficial dose and regrowth of the hair occurs after 2 or 3 months — wigs should of course be provided before the depilation occurs. The dosage of Dexamethasone is reduced to a maintenance dose of 2 mg daily during the treatment. Although a complete remission of symptoms and signs is rare, a return to restricted activity can be expected although ultimate resumption of full work is impossible.

Choroidal metastases
Bilateral choroidal metastases are not uncommon and since they result, if untreated, in blindness, treatment is of great importance. Local irradiation produces shrinking of the deposits, arrests the further extension of retinal detachment and produces considerable improvement in residual sight. Both eyes may require treating and a fairly large dose (4500 rad in 3 to 4 weeks) is necessary. Where the disease is slowly progressing and lengthy survival expected, care must be taken not to produce cataract by irradiation of either lens.

Abdominal disease
Control of abdominal disease is most importantly by hormone therapy combined with chemotherapy, but radiotherapy may prove of value in the treatment of ascites and in any site where there is pressure from localised disease. Ascites is best controlled by paracentesis and chemotherapy, but where these are ineffective the intraperitoneal injection of colloidal solutions of radiogold, radiophosphorus or radioyttrium may be of value — the choice depending upon the estimated dimensions of the deposits. As in the treatment of pleural effusions chemotherapy, the simplest treatment, is to be preferred.

Hepatic metastases seldom respond sufficiently to produce even symptomatic relief, but radiotherapy should be considered where there is a localised painful deposit and also in cases where obstructive jaundice is caused by pressure on the bile duct. Similarly local irradiation may be of value where masses of glands produce obstruction of the duodenum or small intestine.

Irradiation of ovaries
Irradiation of the normal ovaries to a dosage of 1500 rad in a week will, after 2 or 3 months, produce a response estimated to

be similar to that produced by oöphorectomy and is therefore often used as part of "hormone therapy" in cases where a rapid response is not considered necessary.

Summary

While radiotherapy as a locally acting agent can only be locally useful in the treatment of widespread carcinoma, it is often of inestimable value to the individual patient in relieving localised symptoms and so prolonging the period of her restricted, but essentially normal, existence in the family and in the community.

REFERENCES

1. Calle, R., Pilleron, J. P. and Schlienger, P. (1973). Thérapeutique à visée conservatrice des epithéliomas mammaires. *Bulletin du Cancer*, **60**, 2, 217–234
2. Calle, R., Fletscher, J. H. and Pierquin, B. (1973). Bases de la radiotherapie curative des epithéliomas mammaires. *Journal de Radiologie et d'Electrologie*, **54**, 12, 929–938

4

Endocrine therapy — ablative surgery

Ian Burn

It is a remarkable clinical fact that progressive human mammary cancer can be influenced favourably by hormonal manipulation, achieved either pharmacologically or by the more drastic method of endocrine organ ablation. In some instances progressive lesions regress to a point where they are no longer visible or palpable, or the response may be less dramatic. In other patients, still perhaps the majority, no such response occurs, however, and the cancer continues to destroy its host.

The effect of a beneficial response to endocrine therapy is twofold. Offensive lesions regress and apparently heal with amelioration of previously distressing symptoms, and life is prolonged often for years. Unfortunately control of the malignant process is never permanent, and when the tumour recrudesces the rate of growth thereafter is frequently rapid.

The last decade has been profitable in furthering our knowledge of the rationale, scope and benefits of endocrine therapy. There is now a general measure of agreement internationally on the indications for, and sequence of application of, the various methods now available and there are indications that some of the fundamental biological problems concerned are near solution. Four major questions remain unanswered however. Why does only a relatively small percentage of tumours respond favourably? Can a non-responsive lesion be converted to a responsive one? What determines recrudescence after response and can this be delayed or even prevented? Is there scope for more selective endocrine organ ablation than practised hitherto?

These are questions for the future and they provide the challenge for continued laboratory and clinical research endeavour. Before considering the prevailing situation regarding endocrine organ ablation and perhaps speculating on future developments, a short review of its history is relevant.

A German physician, Albert Schinzinger, is generally given the credit for first indicating that human mammary cancer might be ameliorated by removing the ovaries. Hayward[1] relates how Schinzinger put to the 18th Congress of the German Surgical Association in 1889 the suggestion that removal of the ovaries might cause the breast to atrophy and the tumour to become encapsulated in the contracting tissue. The major landmark, however, undoubtedly was the contentious but practical step taken by the Scottish surgeon Beatson in 1895 of removing the ovaries in 2 premenopausal women with advanced mammary cancer. This historic event is described in detail by Hayward[1] in his book. Beatson noticed regression of tumour in both patients, but his observations surprisingly provoked little apparent response from his colleagues of the time.

By 1900, however, sufficient experience of oöphorectomy had occurred for Boyd, a Surgeon at Charing Cross Hospital, to report on the results of the procedure in 54 women, collected from a variety of sources. Boyd[2] reported favourable response in about one-third of the patients. With the advent of practical radiotherapy, it was not long before irradiation of the ovaries was advocated as a satisfactory means of achieving castration. According to Stoll[3], Halberstadter introduced the technique in 1905, and both surgical and irradiation castration have been practised extensively ever since.

The prevailing assumption in the 1940s and 1950s was that the elimination of endogenous oestrogen synthesis was all-important in attempting to control advanced mammary cancer by endocrine methods. Recognition of the contribution made by the adrenal glands in oestrogen synthesis led to courageous attempts by Atkins to treat the disease by subtotal adrenalectomy, at a time when cortisone was not available for subsequent replacement therapy. In his Bradshaw lecture to the Royal College of Surgeons of England, Atkins[4] described how in 1947 and 1948 he carried out 6 operations on women with advanced mammary cancer, in which the whole of the right adrenal gland was removed and approximately $\frac{3}{4}-\frac{7}{8}$ of the left. Definite regression of tumour was observed in 2 patients, but the problems of adrenal insufficiency at that time were prohibitive.

By the early 1950s effective cortisone replacement had become reality, and the culmination of years of remarkable laboratory and experimental animal research occurred when Huggins and Bergenstal[5] reported for the first time successful *total* bilateral adrenalectomy in patients with advanced mammary cancer. The era of practical major endocrine ablation therapy had arrived.

A natural consequence was investigation of the potential of surgical hypophysectomy, as an even greater guarantee of suppression of endogenous oestrogen activity. Luft and Olivercrona[6] were first to publish successful remission of the disease after transfrontal hypophysectomy, a technique soon adopted by other neurosurgeons working in close co-operation with surgical colleagues dealing with the disease.

Although surprisingly little interest appears to have been evinced in developing techniques for irradiating the adrenal glands, considerable effort and ingenuity has occurred in relation to the pituitary. Most of the historical landmarks of the recent past were concerned with this aspect of major endocrine ablation.

External irradiation of the pituitary gland until recently posed considerable problems of confining effective dosage to the gland without damaging vital adjacent structures. For this reason, therefore, considerable effort centred around direct implantation techniques in the 1950s. These efforts were rewarded by the development of a number of alternative techniques.

Forrest and Peebles-Brown[7] described a technique of implanting radon seeds into the pituitary, but there was a high incidence of irradiation damage to local structures. Similar problems occurred with γ-emitter radioactive gold (^{198}Au) when doses sufficiently high to ensure destruction of the pituitary were employed. Various groups of workers eventually showed that the β-emitter ^{90}Y, with a half-life of 2.4 days, provided the most satisfactory method of interstitial irradiation with least risk of severe morbidity. Techniques described and used to this day[8], included the insertion of a screw with a "war-head" of ^{90}Y, and the intrahypophyseal implantation of ^{90}Y seeds through a cannula positioned precisely under X-ray control, the cannula being inserted through a small incision made near the inner canthus[9,10].

More recently, attention was redirected to surgical excision of the gland by routes other than the neurosurgical transfrontal approach. This led to the development of transethmosphenoidal hypophysectomy[11,12]. The procedure, in which a dual approach to the gland is made through the nose and through a small incision near the inner canthus, has been adopted by many otolaryngologists, and with experience has proved to be both safe and generally suitable for adequate removal of the gland.

CASTRATION

It is conventional to regard castration of the female for mammary cancer, either by surgical removal or irradiation of the ovaries, as simple endocrine therapy. Castration is thus placed in the same category as therapy by administration of hormones and the term distinguishes it from major ablation of the pituitary and adrenal glands. It should not be thought that the distinction is necessarily made because of the magnitude of the surgery involved. Rather it relates to the degree of change in hormonal environment caused by the treatment.

It is possible that the relationship of oestrogenic activity to the genesis and inactivation of mammary cancer was over-emphasised in the 1940s. There is no doubt, however, that removal of the ovaries deprives the individual of a major source of endogenous oestrogen supply and may result in dramatic changes in the behaviour of mammary tumours.

Adjuvant castration

The treatment of mammary cancer by castration has been considered in relation to two separate requirements. The first is the delay or prevention of recrudescent disease in women undergoing mastectomy for primary disease; so-called "prophylactic" oöphorectomy. The second is its use as active treatment for recognised advanced disease.

From the outset it is necessary to be clear about one important fact. As with all other forms of endocrine therapy for mammary cancer, there is no reason to presume that the disease is ever eradicated totally by such methods. Control may be achieved for very long periods, even with apparent total disappearance of active disease, but it always recurs. Control is probably achieved by subtle alterations in the kinetics of the cell cycle and future research may enable us to exploit these changes to even greater advantage. For the present, recurrence after even the most dramatic response is a certainty. The term "prophylactic castration" is a misnomer, therefore, and its use should be discontinued. Recurrence after mastectomy with adjuvant oöphorectomy is not prevented, merely delayed.

Hayward[1] reflected that responsibility for almost all the prospective clinical investigative work on the subject rests with Nissen–Meyer of Norway and Mary Cole of this country. The results of these two now classical studies are well-known, and were reported in detail at the First Tenovus Symposium in Cardiff in 1967[13,14].

In Nissen–Meyer's study, 448 women under the age of 70 years with designated Stages 1 or 2 disease were entered in a prospective clinical trial. Patients were allocated randomly into 2 groups. One group had ovarian function suppressed at the time of mastectomy, the other group did not. The method of ovarian suppression in this trial was not consistent, some patients being castrated surgically, others by irradiation. Nissen–Meyer's protocol was a complicated one, perhaps excessively so, involving multiple separate studies of different groups. There was considerable pre-selection of premenopausal patients, those with an adjudged bad prognosis (essentially Stage 2) being excluded from the study. The majority of women in the trial thus were post-menopausal.

Nissen–Meyer's conclusions[13] may be summarised as follows. Adjuvant castration delayed the appearance of recurrent disease in premenopausal patients by about 2 years, but the number of such patients in the trial was small. Post-menopausal patients in the primarily castrated group who subsequently developed further disease had about 1 year longer free-interval than their counterparts in the control group.

Examination of the survival rates is interesting. Stage 1 patients primarily castrated had greatly improved survival in the early years of the trial, but as follow-up progressed the control group showed the better survival. As expected, patients with Stage 2 disease had a much worse survival rate than those with Stage 1. Stage 2 patients primarily castrated had better survival rates throughout the whole period of follow-up than the control group, but in fact the majority of patients with Stage 2 cancers in both groups eventually died from the disease.

Nissen–Meyer made the interesting observation that the beneficial effect of primary castration in post-menopausal women was not confined to the younger women, but occurred equally in patients over 60 years.

Cole and her colleagues also carried out a prospective clinical trial at the Christie Hospital, Manchester, to assess the value of adjuvant primary ovarian suppression. 744 patients were included and Cole has published the results after 10 years follow-up[14]. Although this was a meticulous trial, the method of selection was not strictly random, patients being allocated into castration and control groups according to the month of their birth. The trial also was not confined entirely to patients with primary early cancer, a few having recurrent disease or advanced primary cancers. Only patients who were pre-menopausal or within 2 years of the menopause were included, and ovarian suppression was achieved by irradiation. It is of interest that Cole reported return of menstrual bleeding in 32.7% of patients who were under 40 years and in 10.2% of those between 40 and 45 years.

Cole reported a crude 10 year survival of 46.6% for the castrated group and 41.6% for the controls, a difference which was not significant in statistical terms. When patients with recurrent or advanced primary disease were excluded there was a larger difference in 10 year survival, favouring the castrated patients with 54.9% compared with 47.5% for the controls. In contrast to Nissen–Meyer's findings in post-menopausal patients, Cole reported that benefit in terms of long-term survival was more apparent in patients with negative axillary nodes than in those with involved nodes.

In assessing the effect on the free-interval between mastectomy and recrudescence, Cole reported a definite delay in the reappearance of active disease in the castrated patients. Both the incidence of local recurrence and of metastases at 10 years were reduced. Cole pondered whether this effect was due simply to the postponement of onset or to the eradication of latent metastases. However, the incidences of metastatic disease of 46.1% in the castrated group and 54.5% in the controls suggests that a large proportion of patients in both groups had existing metastases at the time of mastectomy, thus making any subsequent evaluation difficult. The incidences of recurrent local disease, namely 23.2% in the castrated group and 29.7% in the control patients were also surprisingly high for patients with supposedly early operable disease.

Cole also took into account the influence of subsequent hormonal therapy. Women included in the earlier years of the trial showed a greater difference in 10-year mortality in favour of the primarily castrated patients, than did those included in later years. There was in fact no difference in crude 10-year survival between castrated and control groups for those women entering the trial during the last 3 years of the collecting period. Cole attributed this finding to improved survival in the control patients due to pursuance, when indicated, of a more vigorous policy of endocrine therapy than hitherto.

Cole concluded that adjuvant ovarian irradiation (and by implication surgical castration) does appear to improve survival after mastectomy, but that this difference is virtually abolished if vigorous endocrine therapy is used in patients with recurrent and metastatic disease. Cole concluded also that in any group of patients with apparently early disease treated by mastectomy, adjuvant castration does delay the onset of the first sign of "reactivated disease".

These 2 trials have been considered in some detail in view of their undoubted importance and influence. Other authors have presented 5-year recurrence and survival figures which suggested benefit after adjuvant castration, but none of these retrospective analyses carry the authority of the two randomised clinical trials. Retrospective studies have not always favoured castration, however. McWhirter[15] reported identical survival rates in patients with adjudged Stages 1 and 2 disease after mastectomy, with and without adjuvant irradiation castration. In another review, Kennedy and his colleagues[16] reported that a delay before recurrence appeared after primary castration, but that there was no improvement in survival rate.

There are discrepancies in the findings of Cole and Nissen–Meyer, although it is difficult to relate the 2 studies because of the greatly differing protocols. Both trials suggested that such benefit as occurred was in terms of delay of recrudescence rather than improvement in survival *per se*. Cole in particular demonstrated that vigorous application of endocrine therapy *when indicated* is as effective in prolonging life as the use of primary adjuvant castration.

A recent important addition to the existing information is the report by Ravdin and his colleagues[17] of another clinical trial carried out in the USA. In this study, patients under the age of 50 undergoing mastectomy for early mammary cancer were allocated randomly either for immediate oöphorectomy or not. Although the follow-up of many of the included patients was relatively short, there was nothing in the preliminary results which suggested that adjuvant castration improved survival or indeed the free-interval between mastectomy and recurrence.

There is nothing in the available evidence which suggests that suppression of ovarian function ever eliminates active disease permanently and this needs to be reiterated when attempting to decide the present role of adjuvant castration. Other aspects of the management of the disease must also be considered. There is a welcome trend towards selecting more carefully according to the extent of the disease before submitting patients to mastectomy, including the search for occult metastatic disease. Patients in whom radical local treatment is contraindicated because of the presence of occult metastases, even with a small primary cancer, become candidates for immediate *therapeutic* castration if in the appropriate age group. Equally the growing influence of "well-women" health clinics must soon reveal a higher proportion of patients with early eradicable disease in whom immediate castration could confer no benefit.

Taking these factors into consideration there would seem to be no further justification for advising adjuvant castration, either by surgery or irradiation, in patients undergoing mastectomy for early operable mammary cancer.

Therapeutic castration
Stoll[3] in his book discussed in detail the basis of hormonal control in mammary cancer. He emphasised that the significance of oestrogen dependence as a theoretical basis for *all* endocrine control of the disease may have been overestimated. In a thoughtful recent extension of his arguments, Stoll[18] reviewed the current knowledge on mechanisms responsible for respon-

siveness, and in particular the role of oestrogens and prolactin. He concluded that the explanation was unlikely to be any single hormonal relationship or unitary hypothesis. Nevertheless, the suppression of ovarian function in pre-menopausal and early post-menopausal women with advanced mammary cancer may result in marked regression of the disease and periods of remission which sometimes last for years. The response to oöphorectomy is largely unpredictable although the longer the free-interval between mastectomy and recurrent disease, the greater the chance of a favourable response[19]. As pointed out by Stoll[3] and Hayward[1], no correlation has been demonstrated between the degree of clinical response and subsequent quantitative changes in oestrogen excretion. It is now generally agreed that castration should be advised for all pre-menopausal patients and those within a few years of cessation of menstruation, as the initial endocrine therapy for advanced disease. Definitions of advanced disease vary, but the term includes local recurrence after mastectomy, diagnosed metastatic disease and adjudged non-resectable local primary disease.

A beneficial response from castration is not necessarily manifest immediately, even after surgical removal of the ovaries, although sometimes symptoms are relieved dramatically. Objective evidence of response tends to be gradual, but if none is apparent by 3 months then it is unlikely to occur. One of the problems in evaluating realistically the true therapeutic value of castration for advanced mammary cancer has been the varied criteria of successful response. This has led to a wide range of reported remission rates. Nissen–Meyer[20] reviewed 15 series with remission rates varying between 15.2% and 50%. As emphasised by Hayward[1] there is need for international conformity in reporting remission rates and he illustrated the recommendations of the Co-operative Breast Cancer Group at the National Cancer Institute, Bethesda[21] as a useful step in this direction. In making comparisons, a number of factors have to be taken into consideration. These are the proportion of pre- and post-menopausal patients in the series, separation of subjective and objective evidence of improvement, and the distribution of the lesions.

At Hammersmith Hospital we adopted a strict approach to the definition of response. For a Grade "A" response, we require that all lesions present at the time of castration regress and no new lesions appear. A Grade "B" response represents clear regression of most of the original lesion but allows for no improvement of a few lesions or the appearance of a few new ones, but with an overall effect of diminution of disease. Patients who show continued deterioration or who fail to show a Grade A or B response 6 months after castration, are regarded as having failed to respond.

In a recent personal series of 56 patients, which included women up to 5 years after the clinical menopause and who have now been observed for at least 3 years since therapeutic castration, the response rate (Grade A plus B) was 21.5% (12 patients). This compares with a response rate of 27.5% in a much larger (160) personal series of older post-menopausal women treated during the same period with oestrogens. In all patients, castration was carried out surgically. There was no mortality from the procedure.

Within the limitations of differing criteria of response, this response rate would seem to be a realistic one and it is in reasonable accord with the 28% remission rate recently reported by Stewart[19] from the Combined Breast Clinics in Glasgow and Cardiff, and the figure of 20–25% reported by Hayward[1].

The menstrual status of the patients has obvious influence on the response to castration. Fracchia and his colleagues[22] reported a series of 85 post-menopausal patients treated by oöphorectomy of whom only 3 responded. All 3 patients were within one year of the menopause. In Stewart's[19] series of 149 patients, 96 were menstruating regularly at the time of therapeutic oöphorectomy and 39% of these responded. Thirty-four patients were within 2 years of their last menstruation and response rate in this group was 18%. In the 19 patients who last menstruated 2–5 years before oöphorectomy, the response rate was only 5% (1 patient). In my own recent series, 33 of the 56 patients were still menstruating at the time of therapeutic oöphorectomy and 9 (27%) responded. Of the 23 patients who had stopped menstruating, only 3 (13%) responded. In a previously reported series, Fracchia[22] recorded 34.5% remission in patients who were regularly menstruating at the time of therapeutic oöphorectomy compared with 27.3% in patients with irregular menstruation. These results suggest that the chance of beneficial response is reduced appreciably if menstruation has stopped and that very little benefit can be expected beyond the 5-year mark.

Stoll[23] suggested that for post-menopausal patients within 5 years of stopping menstruation, selection for therapeutic castration should be based on cytohormonal evaluation by serial vaginal smears and estimation of urinary oestrogen content. Castration was advised as initial endocrine therapy if levels were persistently high or showed cyclical fluctuation. This method of selection was also advised by Stoll for younger women who had undergone hysterectomy in the preceding 5 years and in whom there was uncertainty whether ovarian activity persisted.

The length of remission in responders varies considerably. Remissions beyond 5 years occur but are exceptional. The mean length of remission in my own recent series is 1 year 11 months, with some patients still in remission. Stewart[19] recorded a remission period of $1\frac{1}{2}$ years in her series of responders. Stoll[23] reported an "average" period of remission of between 10 and 25 months. A patient responding favourably to therapeutic castration may thus expect around 2 years of symptom free life before further treatment becomes necessary.

A final comment is required on the relative merits of surgical and irradiation castration. Nissen–Meyer[13] from his studies concluded that "oöphorectomy was not found superior to ovarian irradiation as a method of primary castration". Cole[14], however, reported return of menstrual bleeding in 32.7% of patients under 40 years of age after ovarian irradiation, and in 10.2% of those between 40 and 45 years. Denoix[24], in a comparative study, found that irradiation of the ovaries produced a more complete suppression of oestrogen activity as measured by the subsequent excretion of gonadotrophins in the urine, than bilateral oöphorectomy.

The situation is somewhat controversial, therefore, and the evidence conflicting. Both methods have their advantages and disadvantages and these have been reviewed in detail by Hayward[1]. My own preference is for surgical therapeutic castration, which provides the opportunity of assessing the extent of metastatic disease within the abdomen and guarantees a more immediate suppression of ovarian function. My policy is to advise oöphorectomy as the first endocrine manoeuvre for all women with advanced mammary cancer who are either pre-menopausal or within 5 years of cessation of menstruation, so long as they are fit enough to undergo the procedure.

Major endocrine ablation

The term major endocrine ablation means removal of the adrenal glands by operation; or destruction of the pituitary by some form of surgical hypophysectomy, the implantation of a radiation source, or a combination of the 2. In favourable situations, major endocrine ablation appears to give the highest rate and longest duration of remission of any of the treatments available for advanced mammary cancer. As with simple endocrine therapy, however, only a proportion of patients benefit from the treatment.

ADRENALECTOMY

The theoretical basis for removal of the adrenals is best sum-marised in the words of Charles Huggins[25] that "the human adrenal gland can secrete sufficient quantities of growth prom-oting steroids to maintain dependent neoplasms". Although not the whole of the story, oestrogen activity clearly plays a role in the progression of mammary cancer. Stoll[3] regards tumours as oestrogen-dependent if castration is successful in causing objective evidence of regression. On this basis relapse of the disease after control by castration has been ascribed to the intact adrenals producing increasing amounts of oestrogen. Bilateral adrenalectomy at this stage might therefore be expected to cause further regression, and this does indeed occur. Adrenalectomy may be successful, however, in causing regres-sion of tumours which previously have failed to respond to castration. In the post-menopausal woman adrenalectomy also causes further regression of tumours which previously have responded to the administration of synthetic oestrogens.

Nowadays the preferred method of bilateral adrenalectomy is by the transabdominal route. The adrenals can be removed with reasonable ease through a single long transverse upper abdominal incision except in patients with marked metastatic hepatomegaly. This avoids the double incision of the posterior route. There is a small mortality from the procedure but this should be minimal with careful selection of patients to ensure their suitability for the operation. There has been 1 death attributable to the procedure among 62 patients recently treated by adrenalectomy on my unit. This was during a period when we returned to the procedure as the preferred major ablation, but selected the patients more rigorously than hitherto according to their fitness to withstand the operation and their chances of obtaining a favourable response. All the operations were done by the abdominal route.

Substitution therapy with cortisone or one of its analogues is essential after bilateral total adrenalectomy but this poses no problems so long as regular follow-up is maintained and the dose increase in times of added stress such as intercurrent infection. A dose of 37.5–50 mg cortisone acetate daily is generally sufficient although some patients also require mineralcorticoid (fludrocortisone) to prevent excessive loss of salt.

The need to remove the ovaries at the time of adrenalectomy has been referred to by Hayward[1]. Most pre-menopausal and immediate post-menopausal patients will already have been castrated as the first method of endocrine treatment for their advanced disease. Hayward implied that concurrent oöphorectomy should be done in all patients with intact ovaries but this is not my own practice in the older post-menopausal women.

In his book, Stoll[3] reviewed the published evidence on rates of response to adrenalectomy, which varied from 28% to 57%. As with assessment of response to simple endocrine therapy, the varied criteria of response makes comparisons difficult. Stoll reported that regression was most likely to occur when lesions predominated in the skeleton and soft tissue, was less likely with pulmonary metastases, and least likely when the disease affected the brain, liver and peritoneal cavity. An overall tumour remission rate in unselected cases of about 30% would appear to be a realistic figure, with an average survival in responders of about 21 months compared with 9 months in non-responders.

DESTRUCTION OF THE PITUITARY GLAND

The importance of the hypothalamic-pituitary axis in the maintenance of mammary tumour growth, through the medium of the pituitary trophic hormones, has been evident ever since Luft and Olivecrona[6] first carried out hypophysectomy for the disease.

The anterior pituitary secretes six hormones, namely growth hormone (GH), thyroid stimulating hormone (TSH), adrenocorticotrophic hormone (ACTH), follicle stimulating hormone (FSH), luteinising hormone (LH) and prolactin. Unlike the first 5 which are *stimulated* by secretion of appropriate releasing factors by the hypothalamus, prolactin secretion is *inhibited*. Radioimmunoassay of the pituitary hormones is now very precise and they continue to be evaluated in detail in mammary cancer[1,3]. Prolactin, which appears to be produced by the erythrosinophyllic cells of the pituitary[26] has a particular role and there is increasing evidence of its ability to influence the rate of growth of mammary tumours. As stated by Hayward[1], the response of human mammary cancer to ablative procedures cannot be explained solely on alterations in circulating levels of oestrogen and androgen, and study of the effects of prolactin activity may provide the clue to better understanding of the phenomenon. Pearson[27] was able to cause reactivation of dimethylbenzanthracene (DMBA) induced mammary tumours in rats, which had regressed following adrenalectomy or hypophysectomy, by the administration of sheep prolactin. The same effect was not achieved by giving bovine growth hormone, oestrogens or progesterone.

Stoll[18] recently suggested, on the basis of a detailed study of a large series of treated patients, that the absolute and relative concentrations of prolactin and oestrogen activity available at the site of a tumour is critical for its response to endocrine therapy. Stoll also suggested that the fact that older postmenopausal women require a relatively lower dose of oestrogen to cause regression of mammary cancer was due to a lower level of prolactin at the target.

Undoubtedly the study of the relationship of prolactin and human mammary tumour growth provides an exciting area of research for the immediate future.

Surgical hypophysectomy
Unlike the adrenals, a number of options are available for destroying the pituitary gland. The various types of surgical hypophysectomy have been described in detail by Schurr[28]. Transfrontal hypophysectomy has remained the choice of the neurosurgeons and this route probably guarantees total destruction of the gland better than any other method.

There has been growing enthusiasm for transethmosphenoidal hypophysectomy, as carried out by the otolaryngologist and which with experience provides very adequate destruction of the pituitary[11,12,29]. As pointed out by Hayward[1] the pituitary stalk is not divided in this operation so that the hypothalamic-pituitary axis may continue to operate between remnants of the gland and the pituitary portal system. Simple section of the pituitary stalk[30], although theoretically having the same physiological effect as hypophysectomy, is rarely practised now as the definitive method of major ablation. It remains a reasonable expedient, however, if there are local anatomical difficulties.

These surgical techniques carry a small mortality and the transethmoidal procedure incurs the added hazard of rhinorrhoea and meningitis. In experienced hands, however, the complication rate is gratifyingly small.

For completeness, mention should be made of the technique of packing the pituitary fossa with wax impregnated with radioactive ^{90}Y after transfrontal hypophysectomy[31]. Although the logic of this refinement is sound, it has not been adopted generally by neurosurgeons.

Irradiation methods
External irradiation of the pituitary has posed considerable problems because of damage to adjacent tissue, although recently proton beam therapy has been shown to be more precise[32]. Although external irradiation of the pituitary has been used infrequently in the treatment of advanced mammary cancer, the same cannot be said of internal irradiation, of which there is now vast experience.

The most popular method undoubtedly has been the use of radioactive ^{90}Y, either in the form of small rods or pellets or attached to the end of a screw inserted and retained in the floor of the sella. The techniques concerned were reviewed in detail by Forrest[33] and the results on large series of patients thus treated have been reported by Juret and his colleagues[34], Forrest and Stewart[8], Sellwood[35], and other authors.

The technique for insertion of the radioactive source has been modified over the years to a point where it now requires only the smallest of incisions near the bridge of the nose, with precise positioning of the isotope into the pituitary under X-ray control. Mortality from the procedure is now rare and the only remaining morbidity of any consequence is the occasional persistent rhinorrhoea which may require a second procedure to seal the defect.

After destruction of the pituitary, by whatever method, patients require cortisone and thyroid replacement therapy. The degree of subsequent diabetes-insipidus varies but most patients require regular pitressin injections in the first few weeks, later replaced by pitressin snuff or nasal spray. After ^{90}Y ablation, most patients surviving beyond a few months require less thyroid and pitressin supplement, and eventually require only cortisone. This is probably a reflection of the failure of the technique to ablate the gland totally and regeneration of partially damaged tissue. Pituitary destruction has the advantage over adrenalectomy that aldosterone secretion is relatively unaffected and post-operative electrolyte imbalance rarely a problem.

Other techniques for destroying the pituitary have been described, such as cryohypophysectomy[36,37] and ultrasonic ablation[38], but to date they have not evoked any widespread enthusiasm.

As with adrenalectomy, the reported response rates after destruction of the pituitary vary considerably. Stoll[3] quoted figures ranging from 12% to 46%, and even higher figures have been reported. During the 4-year period 1966–69 when pituitary ablation with ^{90}Y (rods) was our preferred method of major ablation, we treated 156 patients with advanced disease by the method. Thirty-five patients (22.5%) had a Grade A response, that is objective regression of all lesions and no new ones appearing. A further 21 patients (13.5%) had a Grade B response, that is regression of most but not all lesions. In this series, therefore, there was beneficial response in a total of 36% patients.

From examination of the literature, Kennedy[39] found that the mean survival of responding patients ranged from 22.7 to 28+ months, compared with 6–9.9+ months for non-responders. These figures are very similar to those reported for adrenalectomy and there would seem to be no doubt that life is prolonged in responders to major ablations.

Stoll[3] evaluated the likelihood of response to pituitary destruction according to the site of disease. He reported that the chance of favourable response was greatest for skeletal lesions and somewhat less for disease of soft tissues, liver and lungs. The range of site sensitivity was not as wide as that for adrenalectomy.

PREFERRED MAJOR ABLATION

The Joint Committee on Endocrine Ablation Procedures in Disseminated Mammary Carcinoma of the A.M.A.[40] examined the results of bilateral adrenalectomy and hypophysectomy from 12 North American clinics. 404 patients had undergone adrenalectomy and 467 hypophysectomy. Remission occurred in 31.7 of the former and 31.3 of the latter. Mean survival of responders was 22 months after adrenalectomy and 20.6 months after hypophysectomy. Seemingly there was no difference in results from the 2 procedures.

Atkins and his colleagues[41] investigated the matter by means of a prospective clinical trial. Patients were allocated randomly for either transfrontal hypophysectomy or adrenalectomy plus oöphorectomy. The final results of the trial were published recently[42]. The success rate from transfrontal hypophysectomy was 36% whereas that from adrenalectomy was only 23%. Successful hypophysectomised patients spent 37.1 months in remission compared with 26.3 months after adrenalectomy. The successful patients in the hypophysectomy group lived on average 9 months longer than those who underwent adrenalectomy.

This very important trial demonstrated that in general transfrontal hypophysectomy done by the experienced neurosurgeon carries a marked advantage over adrenalectomy.

The prospective clinical trial is also being used by Hayward and his colleagues[42] to compare transfrontal hypophysectomy with the transethmoidal operation. The results of this and similar studies will be awaited with great interest.

Denoix[24] has concluded that long-lasting objective regressions after pituitary ablation are almost always the result of total destruction of the hypophysis. On the present somewhat crude evidence[8,24] it is clear that implantation irradiation fails to ablate the pituitary completely in at least 30% of patients. Use of more precise methods of evaluating the completeness of ablation will almost certainly show this figure to be too low. My own experience of long-term follow-up after ^{90}Y ablation certainly suggests that the majority of patients are not totally ablated.

It might be expected therefore that ^{90}Y ablation does not achieve such good results as surgical adrenalectomy or hypophysectomy. Certain prospective studies undertaken in this country[43] seem to support this contention. In all these comparisons, however, the skill and experience of the surgeon is at least as important as the type of procedure itself.

The situation concerning the comparative merits of the various methods of major endocrine ablation is by no means clear as yet, but on the available evidence may be summarised as follows. Complete destruction of the pituitary gland in general provides better chance of causing tumour regression than does complete removal of the adrenals. The transfrontal operation provides the best guarantee of total hypophysectomy although this is also possible by the transethmoidal route in experienced hands. Implantation of ^{90}Y into the pituitary, although the simplest of all the methods, is unreliable as a guarantee of total ablation. Adrenalectomy remains a reasonable alternative to ^{90}Y ablation if facilities for surgical hypophysectomy are not available.

All these methods must be recognised for what they are, namely crude destruction of vital tissue to achieve results that undoubtedly in the future will depend upon much more precise ablation of only the implicated portions of the pituitary and probably hypothalamus.

TIMING OF MAJOR ABLATION
The order of application of endocrine therapy has provoked great interest and is of considerable practical importance. While

it is reasonable to try simple endocrine therapy in all patients with advanced disease unless specifically contraindicated, it is a different matter where major ablation is concerned, even though the mortality and morbidity rates from these procedures are now very low.

A disadvantage of using simple endocrine therapy first has been that many patients have deteriorated so much during the preliminary treatment that subsequent major ablation was impossible. Dao and Nemoto[44] reported that 43% of their patients became unfit for major ablation while on androgen therapy.

Dao and his colleagues[45] reported a rather complicated prospective randomised clinical trial in which they compared the results of "primary" adrenalectomy with "secondary" adrenalectomy after previous conventional simple endocrine therapy. Only about half of the latter patients in fact underwent adrenalectomy, but examination of the survival curves of the 2 groups suggested that patients treated by primary adrenalectomy were certainly not at a disadvantage.

More precise information has been provided, however, by 3 prospective randomised clinical trials carried out in this country. Atkins and his colleagues[46] studied 191 patients with advanced breast cancer who had had no previous endocrine therapy, who were treated either by immediate major ablation (adrenalectomy or hypophysectomy) or by simple endocrine therapy and then subsequent major ablation. The survival curves in the 2 groups were remarkably similar. The mean survival was slightly better in the group in which major ablation was delayed although a greater percentage of survival was spent in remission in the patients submitted to immediate ablation[1].

In a similar randomised clinical trial involving 119 patients with advanced mammary cancer, Forrest and his colleagues[47] compared the results of immediate pituitary ablation by the implantation of ^{90}Y with simple endocrine therapy and delayed pituitary ablation. As reported by Stewart[48] there was no statistically significant difference in the survival curves of the 2 groups although the trend was in favour of patients treated initially by simple endocrine therapy, especially among the pre-menopausal patients and patients with advanced local disease.

In a third prospective clinical trial carried out at Hammersmith Hospital, we have also compared the results of immediate pituitary ablation (^{90}Y rods) with delayed ablation after initial simple endocrine therapy in patients with advanced mammary cancer. Patients were randomly allocated to one or other group and included those with advanced local disease, widespread local recurrent disease, and diagnosed metastatic disease. Patients who had received previous endocrine therapy were excluded. The trial was stratified in order to match patients according to the site of disease (osseous only; local only; others) and menopausal status (pre-menopausal; up to 5 years after the menopause; more than 5 years post-menopausal). The simple endocrine therapy varied according to the menopausal status of the patient.

One hundred and thirteen patients were admitted to the trial, 108 of whom were matched. Only the 54 pairs have been considered in the subsequent analysis, which represents the results of the study with a minimum follow-up of 5 years.

(a) Response rate
A complete response to treatment was considered to have taken place if there was clear objective evidence that all lesions had regressed and no new ones appeared. Thirteen of the 54 patients (23%) submitted to immediate pituitary ablation responded, compared with 15 of the 54 (29%) treated first by simple endocrine therapy. Of the 15 responders in the latter group, 6 responded to the simple endocrine therapy alone, 2 to the major ablation alone, and 3 to both forms of therapy. Three patients in this group who responded to simple endocrine therapy died before pituitary ablation could be done and 1 remains in remission. Eighteen of the 54 patients in this combined therapy group died before pituitary ablation could be done.

(b) Survival
The mean length of survival of the responders treated by immediate pituitary ablation was 41 months (4 still alive) compared with 48 months (3 still alive) for those treated first by simple endocrine therapy. The survival curves in the two groups are shown in Figure 4.1. Although the curves appear similar when all patients are considered, there is an obvious trend in

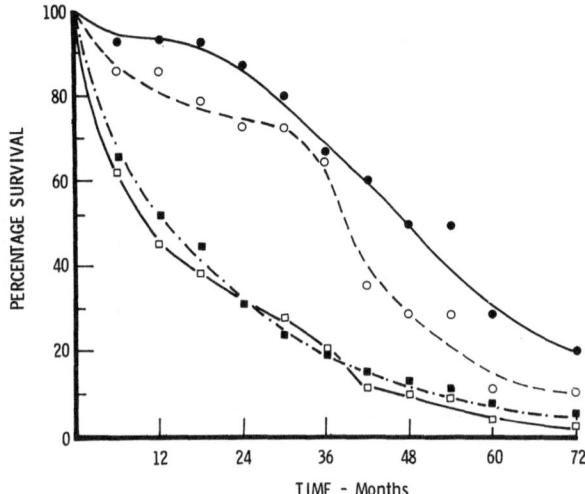

Figure 4.1   Survival curves in Hammersmith clinical trial of timing of major ablation. The lower curves represent survival of all matched pairs in the trial. The top curves represent survival of those patients who responded to endocrine therapy. Responders: ●——● Late ablation; o——o Early ablation. All patients: ■—·—■ Late ablation; □——□ Early ablation

favour of those treated by delayed pituitary ablation when only the responders are considered.

The mean length of survival of the non-responders (all now dead) was the same in both groups, namely $8\frac{1}{2}$ months, emphasising the very worthwhile effect of endocrine therapy in responders.

(c) *Time in remission*   (*Figure 4.2*)
The mean time spent in remission was 30 months for those patients treated by early ablation and 33 months for those receiving late ablation. The percentage of survival time spent in remission was thus 74% and 68.5% after early ablation and late ablation respectively.

None of these differences is statistically significant (at the 0.05% level) and the longer survival after late ablation perhaps has to be weighed against the greater percentage of survival time spent in remission after early ablation.

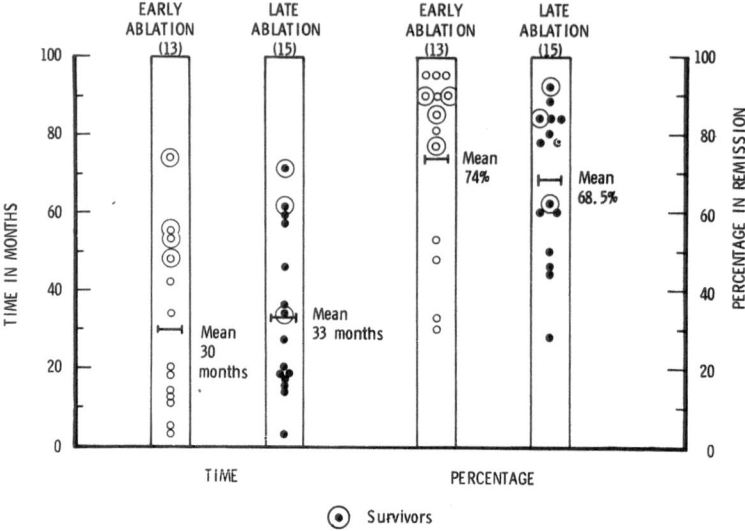

Figure 4.2 Time in remission. The left hand columns show the time spent in remission of the responders in the two groups of patients. The right hand columns indicate the percentage of survival time spent in remission.

The results of this and the previous 2 described trials, carried out in 3 different centres, clearly show that immediate major ablation generally confers no benefit in terms of incidence of response or length of survival. They vindicate the policy of using simple endocrine therapy first, especially in an era when greater selection is being made of patients for major endocrine ablation. It has to be remembered, however, that clinical trials are about groups of patients and do not necessarily decide what is right for the individual. Simple endocrine therapy also should not be persevered with to a point that a patient becomes too ill even to be considered for major ablation.

At the beginning of this chapter, reference was made to 4 major questions concerning endocrine therapy of mammary cancer which require our urgent attention. The last of these 4 questions, namely "is there scope for more selective endocrine organ ablation than practised hitherto?" is of considerable importance if we are to avoid subjecting patients to treatments which are doomed to fail.

Tests of prediction are dealt with in detail elsewhere in this book and there is now every hope of absolute prediction of response to major ablation becoming reality in the next decade. Already with knowledge of the menopausal status of the patient, the free interval between mastectomy and relapse,·the exact distribution of disease, the previous response to simple endocrine therapy and the urinary discriminant function, we are able to make a reasonably accurate prediction of the outcome of major endocrine ablation for any individual patient. Although of undoubted benefit to many sufferers from advanced mammary cancer, no patient should now be submitted to adrenalectomy or hypophysectomy until the above factors have been carefully considered. Where the likelihood of beneficial response is negligible, major endocrine ablation should not be carried out. Equally, where the prediction factors are favourable, no patient fit enough to withstand operation should be denied the appropriate procedure.

REFERENCES

1. Hayward, J. (1970). *Hormones and Human Breast Cancer*. London: Heinemann
2. Boyd, S. (1900). On oöphorectomy in cancer of the breast. *Brit. Med. J.*, **2**, 1161
3. Stoll, B. A. (1969). *Hormonal Management in Breast Cancer*. London: Pitman
4. Atkins, H. (1966). Carcinoma of the breast. *Ann. Roy. Coll. Surg.*, **38**, 133
5. Huggins, C. and Bergenstal, D. M. (1952). Inhibition of human mammary and prostatic cancers by adrenalectomy. *Cancer Res.*, **12**, 134
6. Luft, R. and Olivecrona, H. (1953). Experiences with hypophysectomy in man. *J. Neurosurg.*, **10**, 301
7. Forrest, A. P. M. and Peebles-Brown, D. A. (1955). Pituitary-radon implant for breast cancer. *Lancet*, **i**, 1054
8. Forrest, A. P. M. and Stewart, H. J. (1967). *Major Endocrine Surgery for the Treatment of Cancer of the Breast in Advanced Stages*, p. 89 (Dargent and Romien, editors). Lyon: Simep
9. Talairach, J., Aboulker, J., Tournoux, P. and David, H. (1956). Technique stereotaxique de la chirurgie hypophysaire par voie nasale, suites operatoires, indications thera peutiques. *Neurochirurgie*, **2**, 3
10. Fraser, R., Joplin, G. F., Laws, J. W., Morrison, R. and Steiner, R. E. (1959). Needle implantation of yttrium seeds for pituitary ablation. *Lancet*, **i**, 382
11. Reed, P. I. and Pizey, N. C. D. (1967). Trans-sphenoidal hypophysectomy in the treatment of advanced breast cancer. *Brit. J. Surg.*, **54**, 369
12. James, J. A. (1962). Surgery of the hypophysis. *Brit. Med. J.*, **2**, 332
13. Nissen-Meyer, R. (1968). *Prognostic Factors in Breast Cancer*, p. 139. (Forrest and Kunkler, editors). Edinburgh and London: Livingstone
14. Cole, M. P. (1968). *Prognostic Factors in Breast Cancer*, p. 146. (Forrest and Kunkler, editors.) Edinburgh and London: Livingstone

15. McWhirter, R. (1957). Some factors influencing prognosis in breast cancer. *J. Fac. Radiol.*, **8**, 220

16. Kennedy, B. J., Mielke, P. W. and Fortuny, I. E. (1964). Therapeutic castration versus prophylactic castration in breast cancer. *Surg. Gynec. Obstet.*, **118**, 524

17. Ravdin, R. G., Lewison, E. F., Slack, N. H., Dao, T. L., Gardner, B., State, D. and Fisher, B. Results of a clinical trial concerning the worth of prophylactic oophorectomy for breast carcinoma. *Surg. Gynec. Obstet.*, **131**, 1055

18. Stoll, B. A. (1973). Hypothesis: Breast cancer regression under oestrogen therapy. *Brit. Med. J.*, **3**, 446

19. Stewart, H. J. (1970). *The Clinical Management of Advanced Breast Cancer*, p. 12. (Joslin and Gleave, editors.) Tenovus

20. Nissen-Meyer, R. (1965). Castration as part of the primary treatment for operable female breast cancer. *Acta radiol. (Stockh.) Suppl.*, **249**

21. Cooperative Breast Cancer Group (1966). *Clinical Evaluation in Breast Cancer*, p. 275. (Hayward and Bulbrook, editors.) London–New York: Academic Press

22. Fracchia, A. A., Farrow, J. H., De Palo, A. J., Connolly, D. P. and Huvos, A. G. (1969). Castration for primary operable or recurrent breast carcinoma. *Surg. Gynec. Obstet.*, **128**, 1226

23. Stoll, B. A. (1969). Hormonal management of advanced breast cancer. *Brit. Med. J.*, **2**, 293

24. Denoix, P. (1970). *Treatment of Malignant Breast Tumours*, p. 51. London–New York: Heinemann

25. Huggins, C. (1967). *Major Endocrine Surgery for the Treatment of Cancer of the Breast in Advanced Stages*, p. 2. (Dargent and Romieu, editors.) Lyon: Simep

26. Fotherby, K. Personal communication

27. Pearson, O. H. (1967). *Major Endocrine Surgery for the Treatment of Cancer of the Breast in Advanced Stages*, p. 215. (Dargent and Romieu, editors.) Lyon: Simep

28. Schurr, P. H. (1966). *The Pituitary Gland*, Vol. 2, 22. (Harris and Donovan, editors.) London: Butterworth

29. Harrold, B. P., Cates, J. E. and James, J. A. (1968). Treatment of advanced breast cancer by trans-sphenoidal hypophysectomy. *Brit. J. Cancer*, **22**, 19

30. Newsome, J. F., Timmons, R. L., Van Wyk, J. and Dugger, G. S. (1971). Pituitary stalk section for metastatic carcinoma of the breast. *Ann. Surg.*, **174**, 769

31. Edelstyn, G. A., Gleadhill, C. A., Lyons, A. R., Rodgers, H. W., Taylor, A. R. and Welbourn, R. B. (1958). Hypophysectomy combined with intrasellar irradiation with yttrium 90. *Lancet*, **i**, 462

32. Lawrence, J. H. (1967). *Major Endocrine Surgery for the Treatment of Cancer of the Breast in Advanced Stages*, p. 173. (Dargent and Romieu, editors.) Lyon: Simep

33. Forrest, A. P. M. (1959). Radiation hypophysectomy. *Cancer*, **6**, 274. (Raven, editor.) London: Butterworths

34. Juret, P., Hayem, M., Estelin, R., Markovits, P., Sarrazin, D., Lalanne, C. and Pierquin, B. (1969). L'implantation d'Yttrium 90 intra-hypophysaire dans le traitement des cancers du sein a un stade avance. Bilan de 300 interventions. *J. Radiol. Elect. Med. Nucl.*, **50**, 645

35. Sellwood, R. A. (1970). *The Clinical Management of Advanced Breast Cancer*, p. 79. (Joslin and Gleave, editors.) Tenovus

36. Wilson, C. B., Winternitz, W. W., Bertran, V. and Sizemore, G. (1966). Stereo-taxic cryosurgery of the pituitary gland in carcinoma of the breast and other disorders. *J. Amer. Med. Ass.*, **198**, 587

37. Norrell, H., Alves, A. M., Winternitz, W. W. and Maddy, J. (1970). A clinico-pathological analysis of cryohypophysectomy in patients with advanced cancer. *Cancer*, **25**, 1050

38. Arslan, M. (1966). Ultrasonic hypophysectomy. *J. Laryngol.*, **80**, 73

39. Kennedy, B. J. (1965). Hormone therapy for advanced breast cancer. *Cancer*, **18**, 1551

40. Joint Committee on Endocrine Ablative Procedures in Disseminated Mammary Carcinoma (1961). Adrenalectomy and hypophysectomy in disseminated mammary carcinoma. *J. Amer. Med. Ass.*, **175**, 787

41. Atkins, H. J. B., Falconer, M. A., Hayward, J. L., MacLean, K. S., Schurr, P. H. and Armitage, P. (1960). Adrenalectomy and hypophysectomy for advanced cancer of the breast. *Lancet*, **i**, 1148

42. Hayward, J. L., Atkins, H. J. B., Falconer, M. A., MacLean, K. S., Salmon, L. F. W., Schurr, P. H. and Shaheen, C. H. (1970). *The Clinical Management of Advanced Breast Cancer*, p. 50. (Joslin and Gleave, editors.) Tenovus

43. Roberts, M. M. (1970). *The Clinical Management of Advanced Breast Cancer*, p. 54. (Joslin and Gleave, editors.) Tenovus

44. Dao, T. L. and Nemoto, T. (1965). An evaluation of adrenalectomy and androgen in disseminated mammary carcinoma. *Surg. Gynec. Obstet.*, **121**, 1257

45. Dao, T. L., Nemoto, T. and Bross, I. (1968). *Prognostic Factors in Breast Cancer*, p. 177. (Forrest and Kunkler, editors.) Edinburgh and London: Livingstone

46. Atkins, H. J. B., Falconer, M. A., Hayward, J. L., MacLean, K. S. and Schurr, P. H. (1966). The timing of adrenalectomy and of hypophysectomy in the treat-ment of advanced breast cancer. *Lancet*, **i**, 827

47. Forrest, A. P. M., Stewart, H. J., Benson, E. A., Ker, H., Jones, V., Kunkler, P. B. and Campbell, H. (1968). *Prognostic Factors in Breast Cancer*, p. 186. (Forrest and Kunkler, editors.) Edinburgh and London: Livingstone

48. Stewart, H. J. (1970). *The Clinical Management of Advanced Breast Cancer*, p. 73. (Joslin and Gleave, editors.) Tenovus

5

Hormones by administration

J. C. Heuson

Introduction

The hormone dependence of human breast cancer was discovered at the turn of the century by Beatson[1] who reported beneficial effects from oöphorectomy as a treatment of this disease. The clinical value of ovarian ablation was fully confirmed during subsequent years, and both radiation and surgical castration became established therapeutic procedures in operable or generalised breast cancer[2,3].

Concurrently, much interest was devoted to the role of sex hormones in experimental mammary tumours. Thus, oestrogens were found to induce mammary tumours in male mice[4], while androgens were found to suppress breast cancer development in female mice[5,6]. Furthermore, synthetic oestrogens bearing resemblance to polycyclic carcinogens proved inhibitory to the growth of a breast-originated transplantable tumour of the rat[7].

The concept of hormone dependence of breast cancer and the observation of growth-inhibitory properties of sex hormones on experimental mammary tumours lead to the successful trial of androgens[8,9] and oestrogens[10-12] as therapeutic measures in human breast malignancies. Extensive investigations subsequently confirmed their usefulness and delineated their precise clinical indication and adverse effects[13-16]. In the meanwhile, new classes of steroids, progestogens[17] and corticosteroids[18], were introduced. More recently, oestrogen antagonists[19,20] and inhibitors of prolactin secretion were subjected to clinical trials[21-23].

The purpose of this chapter is to describe the use of hormones and hormone-related compounds in the management of breast cancer. Attempts[24] to administer hormones for prophylaxis of recurrences after mastectomy proved disappointing.

113

Therefore, the discussion will be limited to the therapy of inoperable and advanced breast cancer. The various classes of compound will be analysed separately. The presentation follows the chronological order of their introduction, although pre-eminence is given to oestrogens over androgens in view of available evidence for their greater efficacy and less severe side-effects. The criteria of evaluation of the therapeutic effects will be defined first in order to avoid the confusion that often arises between subjective effects and objective responses.

Criteria of evaluation of therapeutic response

Many reports in the literature have been confusing subjective benefits and objective tumour regression. Some classes of hormone are particularly prone to induce subjective effects and clinical improvement, without stopping tumour progression. Thus, androgens often give a feeling of well-being and of improved strength, as well as a decrease in bone pain. Corticosteroids produce similar effects, sometimes to a considerable degree; they may also alleviate respiratory distress and other complications resulting from oedematous and inflammatory reactions around tumour deposits. However, clinical improvement in such cases is often associated with relentless progression of the disease.

Generally hormonal therapy fails to achieve valuable clinical improvement, in terms of quality and duration, unless it produces objective remission. This is defined as a reduction in size of all tumour masses disseminated in the body. Recognition of objective remissions must rely upon methods of clinical evaluation using well-defined criteria. It is also necessary that these methods be standardised in order to allow comparison of the therapeutic effectiveness of various endocrine modalities.

The detailed protocol used by the Cooperative Breast Cancer Group, sponsored by the US National Cancer Institute, fulfills entirely these requirements[25]. It was adopted with minor variations by most investigators in the field[26]. The main points of this protocol may be interpreted and summarised as follows.

Female patients with recurrent, inoperable or metastatic carcinoma of the breast proved by biopsy, are eligible for hormonal therapy if they are more than 1 year post-menopausal or if, after surgical castration, there is objective evidence of advancing disease.* Patients are not eligible, with minor exceptions, if they have already received hormone therapy for their breast cancer.†

Before initiation of treatment, each patient has to undergo a thorough initial work-up. This includes a complete clinical examination with accurate measurement of cutaneous, sub-cutaneous, superficial lymph nodes and breast lesions. Measurement is carried out with a caliper; whenever possible, photographs of superficial lesions are obtained. A skeletal survey will include X-rays of the major bones. Lesions of the thoracic viscera are measured on chest X-rays and tomographs. Pleural effusions and their rate of accumulation are not easily quantified and may not serve as criteria of evaluation. Lesions of the abdominal viscera are assessed mainly by clinical examination. Isotopic liver scanning has recently become a most useful tool in the assessment of hepatic involvement. Brain metastases are difficult to quantify; all methods presently available should be used.

Diagnosis of objective remission is based on the following definition: there should be a measurable decrease of at least 50% of all demonstrable lesions, while the remainder are static‡. A successful response is inadmissible when there is progression of any lesion, appearance of new ones or absence of objective change in any metastatic lesion after 6 months of therapy.

Evaluation requires the repetition of all items of the initial work-up. This is most important because it is not unusual that some visible lesions such as soft-tissue lesions regress during therapy while others progress or new ones appear, as for example in the skeleton. Healing of ulcerated lesions or of bone-fracture, or drying of a pleural effusion cannot be considered as evidence of an objective remission; on the other hand, fracture of a bone already involved or collapse of a vertebra are not definite evidence of progression. Assessment of skeletal lesions is difficult:

---

* Justification for selecting post-menopausal patients will appear further in this chapter.
† This provision is dictated by the investigative purpose of the protocol but is not necessarily justified in therapeutic practice, although consideration should be taken of "withdrawal responses" as discussed later.
‡ Because assessment of osseous lesions is often difficult (see below), remission is acceptable by this definition even when osseous lesions also remain static.

significant recalcification of previously lytic lesions is the only criterion of improvement; disappearance of osteoplastic lesions is also acceptable, but is rarely to be expected.

An important provision of the protocol of the Cooperative Breast Cancer Group is that evaluation of all cases be reviewed by two independent clinicians. This precaution avoids publication of therapeutic results that are biased by the enthusiasm — or pessimism — of the investigator.

In this chapter, the discussion will be restricted mainly to the published studies which were based on criteria similar to those used in the protocol described above. Clinical improvements unassociated with objective remissions, which occur specifically with certain categories of hormones, will be the subject of separate consideration.

Oestrogens

EXPERIMENTAL BASIS AND HISTORICAL BACKGROUND

The use of oestrogens in the treatment of breast cancer has evolved partly from studies on the growth-inhibitory properties of carcinogenic polycyclic compounds and their relationship to synthetic steroids. Haddow[27] observed that certain polycyclic hydrocarbons inhibited growth of the Jensen rat sarcoma and that the growth-inhibitory activity of various compounds was strikingly correlated with their carcinogenic potency. He suggested that carcinogenic substances may act primarily by producing a certain type of inhibition in the activity of the cell. It was also found that certain carcinogenic hydrocarbons displayed oestrogenic activity[28] in addition to growth-inhibitory properties[29]. Further experiments indicated that hydrocarbon derivatives of ethylene, such as analogues of triphenylethylene, which have a carbon skeleton resembling that of polycyclic carcinogens, were oestrogenic compounds that inhibited growth of the Walker rat carcinoma 256, derived from a spontaneous mammary tumour[7]. Diethylstilboestrol is a potent oestrogen belonging to the same family of ethylene derivatives. Potent synthetic or natural oestrogens have well-recognised growth-stimulating properties on specific target tissues; yet, given in large amounts, they inhibit growth, not only of experimental tumours but also of the body[30,31], of normal tissues such as hair[32], testes[33], and even the mammary gland[34]. It is noteworthy that oestrogenic compounds have a carcinogenic action in animals, especially on the latter two tissues[4,33].

Consideration of these experimental data, demonstrating a distinct influence of polycyclic hydrocarbons and related oestrogenic compounds on normal and tumour tissue growth, led Haddow et al.[12] to undertake the clinical trial of synthetic oestrogens in advanced breast cancer. The compounds used in the first trial were triphenylchlorethylene, triphenylmethylethylene and diethylstilboestrol. Indeed, earlier reports on the successful use of diethylstilboestrol in the treatment of prostatic carcinoma[35] also acted as a strong incentive in the first trials of synthetic oestrogens in breast cancer[10,11,36]. Tumour regression sometimes spectacular and complete was described in a fair number of cases, especially with a patient over 60 years of age; except in rare instances, other cancers did not respond. Since the early reports, large series have accumulated, which confirmed the initial results[15,17,37-39].

INCIDENCE OF OBJECTIVE REMISSIONS

Oestrogen therapy of breast cancer has been mostly restricted to post-menopausal women for reasons discussed below. In this category of patient, the incidence of objective regression obtained in four representative studies is given in Table 5.1. A striking feature is the variability of the remission rates reported, which is a common finding in the field of endocrine therapy of breast cancer. It is due to several factors among which are selection of patients, methods of evaluation and sampling

Table 5.1   OESTROGEN THERAPY OF ADVANCED BREAST CANCER IN POST-MENOPAUSAL WOMEN

| Investigator | No. patients | | % |
	Total	Obj. remission	Obj. remission
A.M.A. Council on Drugs[15]	357	134	37
Cooperative Breast Cancer Group (C.B.C.G.)[13]	218	34	16
Stoll[132]	407		31
Kennedy[129]	55	16	29

variations. As an example, analysis of the studies of the A.M.A. Council on Drugs[15] and of the Cooperative Breast Cancer Group[13] (C.B.C.G.) discloses the following factors that may

Table 5.2　INFLUENCE OF INTERVAL BETWEEN MENOPAUSE AND BEGINNING OF HORMONE THERAPY

A.M.A.[15]			C.B.C.G.[13]			Stoll[133]		
Interval (years)	Remissions*	%	Interval (years)	Remissions*	%	Interval (years)	Remissions*	%
0–4	4/32	12	0–5	5/75	7	0–5	4/59	7
5–8	16/42	38	5–10	9/31	29	6–9	7/30	23
9–12	21/57	37	10+	20/112	20	10+	79/299	26
13–16	22/54	41						
17+	46/125	37						

*Objective remissions/No. patients treated

account for the large difference between their results: (1) the C.B.C.G. protocol provides that all patients must have advancing disease; this important provision was not required in the A.M.A. study. (2) The patients in this particular study of the C.B.C.G. seemed to have an unusually poor prognosis: the control group treated with testosterone propionate had an incidence of remissions of only 22/221 cases (10%) in contrast to 112/521 cases (21.5%) in a previous study[14]. These two factors tended to disfavour the C.B.C.G. study, as compared to the A.M.A. study, in regard to oestrogen effectiveness.

FACTORS INFLUENCING OESTROGEN RESPONSE

Age
Already in the early publications[10,11], it appeared that the frequency of objective response was higher in older patients: the reported remission rates were of 14% under 60 years of age, and of 38% at 60 years of age and above. In the A.M.A. series[15], the correlation between age and frequency of response was statistically highly significant ($P < 0.0005$).

Interval after menopause
The influence of the interval between menopause and beginning of hormonal therapy is shown in Table 5.2. The results are concordant and suggest that the likelihood of obtaining a remission is less frequent in the patients within 4–5 years of the menopause, but that it reaches a plateau thereafter.

Pre-menopausal patients
Oestrogen therapy has usually been restricted to post-menopausal women. Reluctance to use oestrogens before the menopause has been based partly on the observation by Pearson *et al.*[40] that physiological doses of oestrogens produced hypercalcaemia in hormone-responsive pre-menopausal women. However, Kennedy[41] reported that massive oestrogen administration induced objective remissions in 4 out of 23 pre-menopausal women. The treatment consisted of diethylstilboestrol, 400–1000 mg/day or sodium oestrone sulphate, 100–800 mg/day, administered orally. Incidentally, all of these 4 patients also responded subsequently to other hormonal therapies.

Hypercalcaemia occurred in 2 patients. These results seem to indicate that there is no fundamental difference between pre- and post-menopausal patients in their capability to respond favourably to oestrogenic compounds.

Site of involvement

There is some difficulty in interpreting the literature with regard to the relative frequency of hormone-induced regressions in the various anatomic sites. This is due to the fact that in

Table 5.3 OBJECTIVE REMISSION FROM OESTROGEN THERAPY ACCORDING TO SITE OF INVOLVEMENT

"Dominant" lesion*	Objective remissions/No. patients treated			
	A.M.A.[15]	C.B.C.G.[13]	Kennedy[129]	Stoll[133]
Soft tissue (breast, skin, nodes)	33/81 (41%)†	11/34 (32%)	6/16 (38%)	75/262 (29%)
Osseous	7/23 (30%)	9/74 (12%)	3/12 (25%)	3/58 (5%)
Visceral	8/25 (32%)	14/110 (13%)	7/27 (26%)	12/68 (17%)

* See definition in text

* In the A.M.A. series, unlike in the others, dissemination is limited to these sites: cases with involvement of multiple systems are excluded

many reports, such as those of the C.B.C.G., the patients are divided into categories according to *dominant* lesions. This means that in case of involvement of multiple systems, the selected category designates the anatomic site whose involvement is associated with the worst prognosis (soft tissue < osseous < visceral). Furthermore, regression of lesions in one system, as for example soft tissue, without change in the osseous lesions is nevertheless accepted as remission in the osseous category.

Some representative results are given in Table 5.3. They should be interpreted with the afore-mentioned qualification in mind. They indicate that soft-tissue lesions are more prone to regress than osseous or visceral ones. This interpretation is correct in so far as the A.M.A. study is concerned because the data refer to patients with unisystemic involvement (see footnote of Table 5.3). In the other series, it is better to state that patients with soft-tissue lesions only are more prone to have an objective remission than those with osseous or visceral lesions as well. In fact, both statements are probably correct in all series, because it is a frequent observation that, in a given patient, soft-tissue lesions may regress dramatically while osseous or visceral metastases progress, whereas the contrary is most unusual. With regard to bone or visceral metastases, the A.M.A. study gives a true estimate of the incidence of regression in these particular sites (see footnote of Table 5.3). It is in good agreement with the study of Nathanson[37], who reported recalcification of bone lesions in 22.6% of 84 patients and regression of lung metastases in 40% of 55 patients. While pulmonary metastases respond fairly well, it is usually agreed that patients with massive liver involvement have a very low incidence of objective response to endocrine measures[42] The same is true for patients suffering from brain metastases.

Free interval
The free interval is defined as the interval between "definitive" treatment of the primary and recurrence of dissemination (or sometimes, initial use of hormone therapy). Analysis of the free interval is complicated by the recognition of a subgroup of patients whose menopause falls *inside* the free interval. In this subgroup the free interval is unusually long, its duration (mean, 87 months, $7\frac{1}{4}$ years) being more than twice that of the other

patients[15]. Whether this particular category is the result of some biological effect associated with the menopause or a mere statistical artifact (the menopause has a greater probability to fall within longer than shorter intervals) is unknown.

In the A.M.A. study[15], the length of the free interval correlated significantly with the incidence of hormone-induced remissions ($P < 0.05$). However, when the privileged subgroup was subtracted from the entire series, the correlation was no longer significant, possibly simply because of the decrease in sample size.

INFLUENCE ON SURVIVAL

Objective remission from oestrogen therapy is associated with an impressively longer survival than absence of remission (Table 5.4). A similar phenomenon has been universally observed, although with quantitative differences, for all types of endocrine treatment. Whether the recognition of objective remissions merely allows the separation of categories of patients with distinctly different prognoses, or whether effective hormonal treatment actually contributes to prolong survival is as yet unsettled. Evidence in favour of such contribution was presented by Huseby[43]; his argument was based on the comparison of survival in his series of treated patients with the survival of patients in a hormonally untreated "historical control" series.

WITHDRAWAL RESPONSE

Withdrawal response, also called rebound regression, has been recognised since the early days of hormone therapy[44]. It consists of an objective remission occurring after discontinuation

Table 5.4 AVERAGE SURVIVAL ACCORDING TO RESPONSE TO OESTROGEN TREATMENT[15]

Status of patients	No. patients	Survival from start of therapy (months)	
All patients	243	16.5	
Regression	87	27.3	$\left.\vphantom{\begin{matrix}a\\b\end{matrix}}\right\}$ $P < 0.001$
No regression	156	10.4	

Table 5.5 WITHDRAWAL RESPONSE AFTER OESTROGEN THERAPY

Author	Response to initial treatment	No. patients	Withdrawal response No.	%	Median duration of withdrawal response (months)	Median survival of responders from onset rebound regression (months)
Huseby[134]	Remission	14	9			
Kaufman and Escher[46]	Remission	39	10	26⎫	7.0	19
	Failure	194	6	3⎭		
Baker and Vaitkevicius[45]	Remission	11	5	⎫		27.5
	Failure	11	2	⎬		
	Inevaluable	3	1	⎭		

of therapy, most often when the latter had been successful. The results of three studies are summarised in Table 5.5. They indicate that rebound regressions are much more frequent after success than after failure of oestrogen therapy. A remarkable observation was that the duration of these responses was only somewhat shorter than the response to the initial treatment[45,46]. Rebound regressions indicated a good prognosis in terms of survival (Table 5.5). They were observed more often in patients with a long free interval[45]. These observations are of interest, first because they show that hormone withdrawal may sometimes be as good a treatment as hormone administration. In this regard, the exact therapeutic value of hormone withdrawal cannot be derived from the data available, because they are from retrospective studies[46], or from studies based on highly selected categories of patients with slowly advancing disease[45]. A second consequence is that the response to a new treatment, if given immediately after discontinuation of oestrogen therapy, especially when it has been successful, is impossible to assess.

PRIMARY vs. SECONDARY OESTROGEN THERAPY

It is generally agreed that previous effective administrative hormonal therapy affects adversely the subsequent responses to other hormones. This was specifically stated by the Cooperative Breast Cancer Group on the basis of experimental evidence[25]. Stoll[47] reported an oestrogen-induced remission rate of 11% in 46 patients previously treated with androgens, contrasting with a 31% remission rate for primary oestrogen therapy. The influence of previous therapy cannot, however, be accurately assessed from the data available. The important point is that secondary treatment does indeed produce remissions and should be attempted unless rapid progression in vital organs requires the use of chemotherapy. It is noteworthy, and probably of great biological significance, that after an initial regression and subsequent reactivation, a second interval of objective regression may be obtained with hormones of the *same* as well as of the opposite type[15]. An illustrative case who experienced 4 consecutive additive and withdrawal responses with diethylstilboestrol has been reported[45].

Oestrogens as well as other steroids, are seldom effective

after major ablation procedures. After adrenalectomy, oestrogens induced 4 remissions in 37 trials whereas cytotoxic chemotherapy produced a 31% remission rate in 82 trials[48]. After hypophysectomy, oestrogens induced 1 remission in 12 patients treated[49]; a combination of oestrogen–progestin produced objective regressions in 2 out of 4 patients who had relapsed after hypophysectomy[135]. These data are of biological interest and may be of therapeutic interest as well in selected cases.

MECHANISM OF ACTION

The therapeutic effect of oestrogens in breast cancer raises a classical, yet unsolved dilemma. It is generally believed that the endocrine ablative procedures (ovariectomy, adrenalectomy) produce breast cancer regression by suppression of the endogenous sources of oestrogens. In this regard, evidence implicating oestrogens rather than other ovarian or adrenal hormones was provided by Pearson et al.[40] who showed that in patients who improved after oöphorectomy, administration of oestrogen in physiological doses (ca. 0.15 mg of ethinyl oestradiol daily) induced reactivation of tumour growth, as evidenced by the development of hypercalcaemia. It appears therefore paradoxical that administration of oestrogens can likewise achieve breast cancer regression.

It is outside the scope of this paper to discuss the abundant but inconclusive literature pertaining to this apparent paradox. The reader is referred to recent reviews of the relevant literature[47,133]. Suffice it to say that it is often admitted that "physiological" doses of oestrogens contribute to the maintenance of growth of oestrogen-dependent breast cancers, while large "pharmacological" doses are inhibitory. It is worth mentioning that a commonly held hypothesis ascribing this inhibitory effect of high-dosage oestrogen therapy to suppression of pituitary prolactin release[51-53] has recently been refuted[54,55]; thus, it was found by radioimmunoassay that oestrogens stimulated rather than inhibited prolactin release in post-menopausal breast cancer patients. Another interesting question that recently received a partial answer is whether patients responding to ablative procedures and to oestrogen additive therapy are the same. Evidence in favour of their identity is provided by the observation that most responders to either modality are those whose tumours contain tissue-specific oestrogen receptors[56-58].

Histological changes that are associated with oestrogen-induced breast cancer regression were carefully studied by Emerson *et al.*[59]. Regression was preceded by simultaneous loosening of the stroma and necrobiosis of the malignant cells, characterised by swelling of the cytoplasm which became pale and vacuolated, and later disintegrated; the nuclei became karyolytic or pyknotic. Whether the tumour cells were affected directly, or secondarily by way of stroma changes could not be established. Subsequently, collagen formed again in the regressive areas and produced tumour-free scars of increased density. Of great importance is the fact that there was also visual proof that some isolated malignant cells, presumably the source of later reactivations, survived even in extensively regressed tumours.

SIDE-EFFECTS OF OESTROGEN THERAPY

Although most systemic effects occurring during therapy are the expected results of the physiological properties of the hormone given, they are regarded as side-effects by the clinicians who use it in breast cancer patients. Side-effects of oestrogen therapy were carefully recorded and analysed by Kennedy and Nathanson[16] in a series of 235 cases treated in a collaborative study sponsored by the A.M.A. Committee on Research. Stilboestrol was used in most patients, usually at a dose of 15 mg per day orally. Equivalent dosages of other natural or synthetic oestrogenic hormones were used, with similar types and incidence of side-effects.

Gastro-intestinal symptoms
58% of the patients had variable degrees of nausea, and vomiting occurred in 38%. With careful attention to the management of these symptoms and adjustment of dosage, the patients usually became tolerant to full dosage. Discontinuation of medication was necessary in less than 10% of the cases, because of severe anorexia, nausea and vomiting. The incidence of these symptoms decreased strikingly with advancing age; thus, nausea and vomiting occurred respectively in some 85 and 65% of the cases at 30 years of age, and only in about 35 and 18% of

the cases at 70 years of age. Anti-emetic drugs may be tried to control symptoms. Phenothiazine derivatives should preferably be omitted on theoretical grounds, because they are potent stimulators of prolactin secretion and thereby induce hormonal imbalance of unknown consequence.

Sodium and water retention
Oedema due to sodium and water retention was observed in $\frac{1}{3}$ of the patients early in the course of therapy. It was much more common with advancing age, reaching a 60% rate at 80 years of age. It varied from mild to massive. Many additional patients had retention of fluid that was not clinically apparent, but could be demonstrated by observing a rapid increment of body weight amounting from 2.3 to 4.5 kg. Existing lymphoedema of the arm on the affected side was frequently exaggerated. 9% of the patients developed congestive heart failure, with resulting death in 2.6%.

Although potentially dangerous, this complication is usually readily controlled by a low-salt diet and, when necessary, the use of diuretics. Great caution should be exercised in elderly patients as well as in those with known cardiac disease.

Uterine bleeding
Vaginal bleeding occurred in 33% of the patients and withdrawal bleeding in 42%. Bleeding during therapy often consisted of spotting or staining for brief intervals. It was more frequent and profuse in young women than in elderly ones and withdrawal bleeding occurred almost invariably. Bleeding during therapy could often be controlled by sharply increasing the dose. The incidence of bleeding markedly increased with prolongation of therapy. Curettage was rarely deemed necessary.

Breast alterations
Pigmentation of the nipples occurred in 80% of women treated. It varied from a faint discolouration to deep brown, frequently associated with a thick, dark, waxy coating. In addition to the nipples, the pigmentation usually involved the areola, with a sharply demarcated border. Pigmentation also involved the axillae and other areas of the body that are usually affected during pregnancy.

Tingling or tenderness of the nipples, engorgement or venous dilatation occurred in some 20% of all cases, usually in younger women.

Urgency of micturition and incontinence
Frequency and urgency of micturition, sometimes associated with incontinence of the stress type occurred in some 25% of the cases. These symptoms were sometimes quite distressing.

Increase in libido
This symptom, unlike that with androgens was rarely encountered.

THE SPECIAL CASE OF HYPERCALCAEMIA

Hypercalcaemia may occur with either oestrogens or androgens during treatment of breast cancer patients with osseous involvement, most often at the time of initiation of therapy. Because hypercalcaemia occurs spontaneously in about 12% of such patients[16], it should not always be ascribed to the treatment. Nevertheless, when induced by hormones, this complication is often more serious and may be lethal.

According to Kennedy and Nathanson[16], hypercalcaemia was observed more rarely with oestrogens than with androgens, the corresponding rates being 2 out of 235 patients and 7 out of 82 patients; these are minimal figures, because calcaemia was not measured in each case.

Induction of hypercalcaemia has often been interpreted as evidence of exacerbation of tumour growth by the hormone[40]. This interpretation has not been firmly established and there is clinical evidence against it. Thus, in a series of 13 patients who developed hypercalcaemia at initiation of oestrogen therapy, 6 could be maintained on treatment for 2 months and 3 of them switched over to positive calcium balance and eventually obtained objective remission of their disease[60]. This suggests that induced hypercalcaemia indicates sensitivity to steroid, but this sensitivity may just as often predict a good response as a detrimental one. It is proposed as a hypothesis that hypercalcaemia may result from loosening of bone matrix near tumour cells comparable to the stromal loosening which was described in primary breast cancer showing signs of regression under oestrogen therapy[59] (see under Mechanism of action).

Even if hypercalcaemia may forebode a favourable response to treatment, it should not be forgotten that this complication is a dangerous one, when hormonally induced, and is often associated with a poor prognosis[61,62].

COMPOUNDS AND DOSAGES
Various oestrogenic compounds have been used with success. The most commonly used are ethinyl oestradiol, 3 × 1 mg daily, and diethylstilboestrol, 3 × 5 mg daily; both are given orally. There is some uncertainty as to optimal dosage: while lower doses are undoubtedly active, there is evidence that the doses recommended here, or even larger in occasional cases, are more effective. Huge doses have been used in pre-menopausal patients, without unacceptable toxicity, as mentioned before; it should be stressed, however, that stilboestrol at the dose of 5 mg daily was reported to increase death from cardiovascular complications in men treated in the same manner for carcinoma of the prostate[63].

Androgens

EXPERIMENTAL BASIS AND HISTORICAL BACKGROUND
Lacassagne and Raynaud[5] administered huge doses of testosterone propionate (2 mg per week) to female R3 mice, a strain with a high incidence of "spontaneous" breast cancer, starting at 1–20 days of age, and continuing for the life-time. No breast cancer was detected in 8 mice surviving more than 6 months while it was expected to show up in 60–70% of the animals. The mechanism was quite obvious since the mammary tissue failed to develop and pregnancy did not occur. At the same time, Nathanson and Andervont[6] reported a beautifully-conducted trial on C3H mice, a strain with a 95% incidence of breast cancer. After a first pregnancy, mice were allocated to two comparable groups of 20. The group treated received 1.5 mg testosterone propionate weekly for a period of 4 months. Only 30% developed breast cancer as compared with 100% in the control group. In contrast to its preventive effect, it was also found that testosterone propionate did not influence growth of

established tumours. In this experiment, unlike that of Lacassagne, testosterone actually prevented the development of
cancer in mammary glands already fully developed.

On the basis of these early animal experiments, androgens
were tried with some success as a palliative treatment of
advanced breast cancer by Loeser[8] and by Ulrich[9] independently, and later by Fels[64]. Farrow and Woodard[65] observed an elevation of the blood and urinary calcium in 3 out
of 3 cases of breast cancer metastatic to bones, and in 2 out of 3
such cases receiving oestrone; hormones had no effect on calcium metabolism in two cases without skeletal metastases (this
is the first report describing induction of hypercalcaemia by
hormones in breast cancer patients with osseous involvement).
Adair and Herrmann[66] using larger doses over longer periods
reported objective response in a few patients in a small group
with advanced breast cancer. After these first attempts, larger
series of breast cancer treated with androgens have accumulated (for review, see Nathanson and Kelley[38]).

INCIDENCE OF OBJECTIVE REMISSION

A precise assessment of the rate of objective remission induced
by androgens can be derived from the large series reported in
the Cooperative Study reported by the A.M.A. Council on
Drugs[15] and in the study of the Cooperative Breast Cancer
Group[14] (C.B.C.G.). Both studies were based on the use of
rigid criteria for evaluation of objective remission. In the former,
patients having received previous treatments were accepted,
whereas in the latter, only previously untreated patients were
eligible for protocol therapy. There was another major difference between these trials: in the first, both pre- and post-
menopausal patients were treated; in the second, only women
with advancing disease after a natural or surgical menopause
were admitted in the trial. Most patients received testosterone
propionate (TP) intramuscularly, 100 mg three times weekly,
although in the A.M.A. series, some of the 415 TP-treated
patients received smaller or larger doses and 165 patients
received other steroid preparations at dosages judged equivalent to TP, 100 mg three times, weekly.

In the A.M.A. study, the remission rate in 160 pre-
menopausal women was 20%, and in 420 post-menopausal

patients, 21.9%. In the C.B.C.G. trial, it amounted to 21.5% in 521 post-menopausal women. It is remarkable that the remission rates were almost identical in these two large series of post-menopausal women. The median duration of remission, in the C.B.C.G. trial was 36 weeks from start of therapy in the 105 patients for whom information was available.

FACTORS INFLUENCING ANDROGEN RESPONSE

Menopausal age
Pre-menopausal patients may respond to androgen therapy, although the incidence of remission is probably much lower than after oöphorectomy. In post-menopausal patients, the interval between menopause, whether natural or surgical, and initiation of therapy has a strong bearing on the success of the latter. The correlation between menopausal interval and remission rate was found highly significant in the A.M.A. series. The influence of the menopausal interval in the A.M.A. and C.B.C.G. studies is given in Table 5.6; the results show that longer intervals are associated with higher remission rates, although a plateau is reached at intervals larger than 5–8 years.

Site of involvement
The results of androgen therapy according to site of involvement are shown in Table 5.7. In the C.B.C.G. series, the remission rate was significantly higher in the soft tissue category than in the other ones; such a difference was not apparent in the A.M.A. study. However, it should be stressed that the categories are not defined in the same manner (footnote of Table 5.7) and should not, therefore, be interpreted similarly (see section on Oestrogen Therapy).

Free interval
The influence of this factor has been assessed in the A.M.A. study. The definition of the free interval as well as the division of the patients into three categories according to the position of the menopause with regard to the free interval has been described and discussed in the section on oestrogen therapy. As with oestrogens, there was a significant correlation between incidence of androgen-induced regressions and increasing

Table 5.6 INFLUENCE OF MENOPAUSAL INTERVAL ON RESPONSE TO ANDROGEN THERAPY

A.M.A.[15]			C.B.C.G.[14]		
Interval (years)	Remissions§	%	Interval (years)	Remissions§	%
0–4	27/154	17.5	1 year	8/92	8.7
5–8	8/61	13.1	1–5	17/100	17.0
9–12	18/68	26.5	5–10	21/82	25.6
13–16	9/38	23.7	10+	66/247	26.7
17+	19/60	31.7			

§ Objective remissions/No. patients treated

Table 5.7 OBJECTIVE REMISSION FROM ANDROGEN THERAPY ACCORDING TO SITE OF INVOLVEMENT

A.M.A.*[15]			C.B.C.G.[14]		
Site of† involvement	Remissions No.§	%	Dominant‡ site	Remissions No.§	%
Soft tissue	16/69	23.2	Soft tissue	40/127	31.5
Osseous	39/162	24.1	Osseous	35/189	18.5
Visceral	10/35	28.6	Visceral	27/205	18.0

* Pre- *and* post-menopausal patients
† Dissemination limited to these sites
‡ Site of "dominant" lesion; if several sites involved, category was selected according to site associated with the worse prognosis (soft tissue < osseous < visceral)
§ Objective remissions/No. patients treated

length of free interval. When the patients were divided into categories according to the menopause, the influence of the free interval on the chances of response remained predominant, particularly in the category associated with an unusually long free interval.

INFLUENCE ON SURVIVAL

As with oestrogens and other endocrine therapies, patients experiencing an objective remission from androgens have a remarkably longer survival than non-responders. In the A.M.A. series, the *average* duration of life for all 427 patients receiving androgens as the only form of steroid therapy was 11.4 months from initiation of treatment. This period of average longevity was of 19.1 months for those patients who demonstrated regression, and only 9.7 months in the non-responsive patients.

In the C.B.C.G. study, the *median* survival time of the remitters was 23 months as compared to only 9 months for the total group. This impressive improvement of prognosis in case of remission was found in all three categories by site of "dominant lesion".

Interpretation of this treatment effect has been discussed in the section on Oestrogen Therapy.

WITHDRAWAL RESPONSE

Withdrawal response or rebound regression, is a frequent occurrence after oestrogen therapy. It also occurs after androgen treatment, but is less frequent. It was observed in 10.1% of 49 trials in patients who initially responded to androgens and later relapsed, and in only 1.2% of 322 trials after androgen failure[46].

SECONDARY ANDROGEN THERAPY

As with oestrogens, androgens are capable of producing objective remission at the time of relapse after a successful course of another steroid, although with less frequency than with primary androgen therapy[15,47]. Androgens may also induce remissions after failure of other steroids. They have also been reported to induce occasional regression of reactivated tumours after oöphorectomy or even major ablative procedures[47].

SIDE-EFFECTS OF ANDROGEN THERAPY

"Side-effects" of androgens are usually manifestations of their normal physiological properties. Some are beneficial but most are adverse because of their intensity and occurrence in the opposite sex. The most dreaded are virilisation and increased libido. Side-effects of androgens were carefully analysed by Kennedy and Nathanson[16] in a work already discussed in the section on Oestrogens. The following is a summary of their observation on 82 patients treated.

Hoarseness

Hoarseness, which was the commonest of the masculinising phenomenon resulting from androgen therapy, occurred in a minimum of 61% of the patients. The incidence increased with prolonged or more intensive therapy. The changes varied from slight huskiness to a coarse, deep, masculine voice. These changes result first from oedema and injection, and later from hypertrophy of the vocal cords. In the majority of the patients, discontinuation of the male hormone was followed by a gradual return of an essentially normal voice. In others, the voice failed to return to pre-treatment quality, due to persistent hypertrophy of the vocal cords.

Hirsutism

Hirsutism occurred in at least 52% of the patients. Its degree was variable. With intensive and prolonged treatment it usually increased and simulated a typical masculine distribution. Extreme hypertrichosis, characteristic of masculinising tumours, was also observed. The presence of increased hair, especially on the face, disturbed many women, especially those having a dark complexion. Hypertrichosis, as a rule, gradually disappeared after discontinuation of therapy.

Alopecia

Partial loss of scalp hair, often associated with hypertrichosis elsewhere, was noted in 22% of the patients. The hair of the scalp became dry and coarse and fell out whenever it was combed. Recession at the temples was noted in some patients, and occasionally baldness of the vertex resulted. It has been suspected that androgens produce alopecia primarily in persons who have a hereditary susceptibility to baldness. When use of the hormone was stopped, hair normally reappeared.

Dermatological changes

Aesthetically distressing was the appearance of acne. The lesion varied from small milia and scattered papules to extensive furuncles and papules over the face, back and chest. Also oiliness and thickening of the skin was noted. Discontinuation of therapy was usually followed by remission of these complications.

Ruddy complexion

The complexion of patients treated over long periods became ruddy and flushed, sometimes resembling the face of patients with Cushing's disease. Ruddy complexion occurred in almost half of the patients. In a substantial number of patients, haemoglobin values rose from subnormal or normal levels to those as high as 19 g per 100 ml, while the cell count and hematocrit rose in parallel.

Increased weight and well-being

One of the most consistent effects was a feeling of well-being, which was recorded in 76% of the cases. Patients depressed and debilitated often became euphoric. Not infrequently, patients bedridden by pain and debility, particularly from osseous lesions, became rehabilitated, even when X-ray examination revealed progression of the disease. Some patients gained so much weight that they became obese, dyspnoeic and generally uncomfortable. At times, it was necessary to give a reducing diet during androgen therapy.

Increased libido

After some months of androgen therapy, 37% of the patients showed an increase in libido; the incidence increased with prolonged therapy. This may not represent the true incidence, since some patients were reluctant to discuss it even after direct questioning. Married women were emotionally less disturbed than widows or spinsters. Some found the change so unpleasant that use of the hormone was discontinued. Clitoris enlargement was recorded in many patients.

Extracellular fluid retention

This complication has been described in the section on oestrogens. It occurs less often than with oestrogens in young women, but with the same frequency in the elderly.

Hypercalcaemia

Induction of hypercalcaemia, its mechanism and prognostic significance were discussed in detail in relation with oestrogen therapy (see section on oestrogens). It was mentioned that hypercalcaemia seems to occur more frequently with androgens than with oestrogens.

COMPOUNDS AND DOSAGE

Testosterone propionate was the first androgen used in the therapy of breast cancer. Subsequent experience indicated that the most effective means of giving testosterone propionate was 100 mg in oil intramuscularly 3 times weekly[25]. It has been administered in this manner in the large studies of the A.M.A.[15] and of the C.B.C.G.[14]. The side-effects of this therapy with special reference to virilising activity were analysed above.

Extensive investigations were conducted, especially by the C.B.C.G.[13,25], in an attempt to find androgen derivatives with greater therapeutic effectiveness and less virilising properties than testosterone. Fluoxymesterone (Halotestin, Ultandren = 9α-fluoro-11β-hydroxy-17α-methyltestosterone) was found effective by the oral route, at a daily dose of 20 mg, producing a remission rate of 15% in 160 patients[13]. As other 17α-alkylated steroids, this compound increases Bromsulphalein (BSP) retention[67] although cholostatic jaundice was only infrequently reported[68]. 2α-Methyldihydrotestosterone propionate (Dromostanolone, Masteril = 4-5α-dihydro-2α-methyltestosterone) given intramuscularly, 100 mg 3 times weekly, was another interesting compound. The response rate (39/193 = 20%) and pattern of response were similar to those with testosterone propionate but virilisation was considerably less when evaluated by the double-blind technique[13]. A similar remission rate was obtained when the compound was given orally as the non-esterified alcohol (150 mg daily)[13].

Δ1-Testololactone is an extremely interesting compound because it is practically devoid of hormonal or metabolitic activity as well as of side-effects. In the early studies, it was given intramuscularly, 100 mg 3 times weekly. The remission rate was similar to that obtained with androgens[69]. There is some evidence suggesting that Δ1-testololactone is active in the same patients as regular androgens[70]. Δ1-Testololactone was found effective when given orally. The optimal dosage of 1 gm daily induced a remission rate of 18% in 115 patients[71]. Side-effects were not analysed in the latter study.

Finally, Calusterone (7β, 17α-dimethyl-testosterone) was reported to induce an unusually high remission rate of 51% either as primary or secondary treatment (41 and 49 patients respectively)[72]. The compound was given orally, 200 mg daily.

Although androgenicity was weaker than with other androgens, some degree was noted in all patients who received Calusterone for more than 12 weeks. 28% of the patients had nausea, intractable in 4%. Nearly all had marked elevation of the BSP retention without jaundice or evidence of liver damage. These remarkable results were not entirely confirmed by the C.B.C.G. in a comparative controlled study: the remission rate was only 28% in 109 patients treated with Calusterone as compared to 18% of 115 patients treated with Δ1-testololactone[71].

Progestogens

PROGESTERONE
Parenteral administration of progesterone, at doses ranging from 100 mg 3 times weekly to 250 mg daily, was reported to produce occasional, short-lasting remissions in breast cancer patients[73,74]. However, huge oral doses (2 g daily) failed to induce a single remission in 29 patients, although definite evidence of pharmacologic activity of this dosage was demonstrated[25].

SYNTHETIC PROGESTATIONAL STEROIDS
17α-Hydroxyprogesterone caproate (Delalutin, Proluton Depot, Primolut Depot), like progesterone itself, induced only occasional remissions[13,75,76].

Interestingly, Delalutin (1 g i.m. weekly) was reported to induce remissions when given together with an oestrogen, after failure of a course of the oestrogen alone[77]. Remission occurred in 6 of 22 patients so treated. However, critical appraisal of this work casts doubt on the author's conclusion. These remissions need not be ascribed to the combination of hormones, but could well have resulted from the administration of either one alone. Subsequent studies of combinations of oestrogens and progestogens gave remission rates that are of the same order as those with oestrogens alone[78-82]. It is concluded that there is no evidence as yet suggesting that progestogens enhance the therapeutic efficacy of the oestrogens.

In contrast to progesterone and to the weak progestogen Delalutin, several more potent progestational agents were found to induce essentially the same rate of remission as reference androgens[13,25]. The principal compounds and dosages used were:

9α-bromo-11-β-ketoprogesterone (Braxorone), 200–2400 mg p.o. daily[83,84].

17α-ethinyl-19-nortestosterone (Norethisterone) and its acetate, 40–60 mg p.o. daily[25,85].

17α-ethinyl-17β-hydroxy-$\Delta^{5(10)}$-estrene-3-one (Norethynodrel), 40 mg p.o. daily[25].

6α-methyl-17α-hydroxyprogesterone acetate (Medroxyprogesterone acetete, Provera), 266 mg p.o. daily[13].

The initial studies have been expanded. Recent reviews confirm the therapeutic value of the potent synthetic progestogens[86-88]. However, their clinical effectiveness cannot be assessed with any accuracy in comparison with the oestrogens or the androgens, in view of the lack of available sizable comparative studies.

FACTORS INFLUENCING PROGESTOGEN RESPONSE

It is difficult to evaluate the influence of age and menopausal status on responsiveness of breast cancer to the synthetic progestogens. Most patients treated were post-menopausal. According to Stoll[47], the vaginal smear has predictive value for the responsiveness to progestogens, given alone or in combination with an oestrogen (Lyndiol): in patients with an atrophic smear, response occurred in only 6%; in those with an intermediate smear, response occurred in 29 or 40% of cases receiving progestogens or Lyndiol respectively.

Progestogens are active as secondary therapy, although it is unclear whether prior response to oestrogens or androgens has a predictive value[84,87,88].

There is some suggestion that progestogens are active mainly on soft tissue lesions and much less so on osseous lesions[47,83,89]. This would not be surprising insofar as a similar trend exists with oestrogen or androgen therapy.

The mechanism of the therapeutic action of progestogens in breast cancer is totally unknown.

SIDE-EFFECTS OF PROGESTOGEN THERAPY

Braxorone was found to produce fluid retention[84] which was often difficult to control[25]. Delalutin (Proluton) exerts the opposite action and actively mobilises oedematous fluid, possibly by competiton with aldosterone[77].

Medroxyprogesterone acetate (Provera) appears virtually devoid of side-effects[87,88,90]; it was not observed to produce oedema, Cushingoid appearance or disturbances of liver function tests[88]. On the other hand, lynoestrenol (17α-ethinyl-17β-hydroxy-4-oestrene) and norethisterone acetate (17α-ethinyl-19-nortestosterone), at doses of 30 and 60 mg respectively, induced hepatic toxicity, involving frequent elevation of the serum transaminase levels, occasional clinical jaundice and histological evidence of parenchymal-cell necrosis in the centrilobular zones[81,88]. In addition, these 17α-ethinyl steroid derivatives produced severe nausea, vomiting and abdominal pain, which necessitated stopping therapy in more than 10% of cases, particularly when given in association with oestrogens as in the contraceptive tablets of Lyndiol (3–6 tablets daily)[81,88]. Other minor side-effects were recorded: breast and pelvic discomfort, dizziness, constipation and rarely breakthrough uterine bleedings[81,88,91].

HYPERCALCAEMIA

Like oestrogens and androgens, progestogens were observed to induce hypercalcaemia. This complication has been reported to occur with the following compounds:

Braxorone, in 3 of 34 patients treated[84].

Medroxyprogesterone acetate, in 4 of 17 patients with extensive bone metastases[89], and in 2 of 34 patients treated[87].

Norethisterone acetate, in 2 of 28 patients[85].

As already stated, some 12% of all patients with osteolytic lesions from breast cancer will have spontaneous hypercalcaemia during the course of their disease. Nevertheless, the chronological relationships between hypercalcaemia and treatment were striking, especially in the 4 cases reported by Kaufman et al.[89], which strongly suggests a causal relationship. It would appear that the mechanism is related to the intrinsic properties of the progestogens, at least with respect to medroxyprogesterone acetate, rather than to conversion to an oestrogen or an androgen. Such conversion of medroxyprogesterone acetate seems unlikely to occur and this compound appears totally devoid of androgenic or oestrogenic properties[89]. This may not be the case for all progestogens, since it is known that norethisterone acetate is converted to ethinyl-oestradiol to the extent of 1 per 1000[85].

Corticosteroids
RATIONAL BASIS
Corticosteroids have been widely used in the treatment of advanced breast cancer. They have been given alone or in association with cytotoxic drugs in the various recent modalities of combination chemotherapy[92].

They were used first to clarify the question whether the cortisone maintenance therapy given after adrenalectomy was involved in the induction of remissions. In order to answer this question, Segaloff et al.[93] treated post-menopausal patients with maintenance doses of cortisone and did not observe true objective remissions. A majority of patients were subjectively improved and pulmonary lesions regressed, but progression of lesions elsewhere was observed. These findings were confirmed by Dao et al.[94] in a randomised study comparing bilateral adrenalectomy and cortisone maintenance therapy alone. Adrenalectomy induced objective remissions in 44.5% of the patients, while cortisone alone failed to induce true remissions although subjective improvement was noted. These studies indicate that cortisone substitution therapy was not the major factor in the induction of remissions by bilateral adrenalectomy.

Corticosteroids were then used in an attempt to achieve "medical adrenalectomy". The results of this line of investigation will now be discussed.

"MEDICAL ADRENALECTOMY"
As a substitute to the surgical ablative procedure, corticosteroids were administered in order to suppress adrenocortical function. A striking observation is the extreme variability of results, in terms of objective remissions, in the various clinical trials reported. Besides differences in patient selection and criteria of evaluation used, sources of variation were differences in type of steroid and dosage used, menopausal status and, in post-menopausal women, presence or absence of intact ovaries.

The latter factor has been a major issue because it was unclear whether post-menopausal ovaries are still able to secrete oestrogens. The question is still unsettled and relevant evidence will be discussed below. As a consequence, some authors resorted to ovarian ablation, irrespective of age, while others did not.

Another difficulty in the assessment of the therapeutic results of adrenocortical suppression resulted from the confusion between *actual clinical improvement* and true objective remission. All authors were impressed by the frequent occurrence of major clinical improvement (decrease in bone pain, control of hypercalcaemia, alleviation of respiratory distress, restoration of appetite, increase in body weight, feeling of well-being, resumption of normal activities), while careful scrutiny often disclosed objective progression in various metastatic sites. In a minority of cases, objective tumour regression was also observed. These are two distinct features of corticosteroid therapy, which are both of value to the patient but should not be confused.

INCIDENCE OF OBJECTIVE REMISSIONS FROM CORTICOSTEROIDS

Reported rates of objective remission have ranged from zero to about 20%. Thus van Gilse[95] failed to obtain a single case of remission in a careful study of 131 post-menopausal patients receiving either cortisone, 100 mg p.o. daily, or prednisone, 20 mg p.o. daily in 4 equally divided doses. Although measurable decrease of metastatic lesions in some areas occurred in 41 patients of 119 evaluable (33%), *in all of them* progression of disease went on elsewhere. These partial failures may possibly reflect an insufficient dosage of corticosteroids. This explanation is suggested by the study of Stoll[96] who treated 80 patients with prednisolone, 30 mg daily. Objective remissions were obtained in 9 patients (11%). However, the dosage of prednisolone proved critical: in most of these patients, control of tumour growth vanished when the dose was decreased to 20–25 mg daily and was restored by resuming the initial dosage. Other studies reported remission rates of about 20% in patients receiving prednisolone or methylprednisolone at daily doses ranging from 24 to 100 mg[50,97,98]. This review, which is not exhaustive, indicates that corticosteroids in large enough dosage are capable of inducing true objective remissions in breast cancer patients. However, the series are too small to draw definitive conclusions as to the actual incidence of the corticosteroid-induced remission. Furthermore, the quality of the remissions is uncertain, and some reports suggest that their duration is short. Attempts to improve the therapeutic effectiveness of corticosteroids by increasing their dosage are hampered by the resulting generation of unacceptable side-effects[96,98].

CORTICOSTEROIDS ASSOCIATED WITH THYROID HORMONES

In some therapeutic trials, corticosteroids were given in association with thyroid hormones on empirical grounds, "to provide additional inhibition of the hypophysis and prevent myxoedema". Lemon et al.[99,100] reported surprisingly high remission rates, in excess of 50%, with this association. However, a critical analysis of their studies leads to reject many of the alleged remissions, because the criteria of remission were often of a subjective nature, and because many patients received concomitant chemotherapy or radiotherapy, or had been subjected to oöphorectomy shortly before. Gardner et al.[101] reported a 24% remission rate, using the criteria of the C.B.C.G., in 46 post-menopausal patients treated with prednisone, 30 mg daily, and sodium liothyronine (tri-iodothyronine), 50 μg daily. These studies fail to provide evidence suggesting that thyroid hormones may improve the therapeutic effectiveness of prednisone.

CORTICOSTEROIDS ASSOCIATED WITH OVARIAN ABLATION

Finally, suppressive corticosteroid therapy was administered as a complement to oöphorectomy or ovarian irradiation, irrespective of age or menopausal status[102–104]. The results of these studies are difficult to interpret because the criteria of evaluation were not precisely defined and because the respective therapeutic parts of adrenal cortical suppression and of ovarian ablation could not be clearly distinguished.

SPECIFIC CORTICOSTEROID THERAPEUTIC EFFECTS

Many investigators[47] were impressed by the frequent occurrence of major clinical improvement during treatment of advanced breast cancer with corticosteroids. Favourable subjective and objective effects develop rapidly, although they are often short-lasting. Improvement consists of a sensation of well-being and of an increase in appetite and weight. Sedation of bone pains is frequent, with improvement in strength and resumption of more or less normal activities. Myelophtisicanaemia may be improved. Reduction of indurated painful areas around tumour invasion, decrease of lymphoedema of the arm and resorption of metastatic serous effusions, especially pleural and pericardial, are not infrequent. Decrease of painful enlargement of the liver, nausea and jaundice have been reported. Alleviation of respiratory distress, even life-saving, is sometimes obtained. These beneficial effects are in some way related to the anti-inflammatory effects of corticosteroids. They often occur, as already stated, while concurrent growth of metastatic disease is visible. In addition, they may be obtained in non-hormonally dependent tumours. For these reasons, they should not be equated with the true remissions that are induced in breast cancer by endocrine measures including corticosteroid administration.

Effect on hypercalcaemia
Although recalcification of osteolytic lesions has rarely, if ever, been achieved by corticosteroid administration, this treatment is very effective in the control of hypercalcaemia. The mechanism is not fully understood. It involves a decrease of intestinal absorption of alimentary as well as endogenously excreted calcium salts. It is possible that other factors may also be operative. The use of corticosteroids, at doses that need not exceed 30 mg of prednisone daily, has become part of the routine treatment of hypercalcaemia, although other measures are often sufficient. Corticosteroids, however, add their other beneficial effects to their specific action on calcium metabolism. High doses of dexamethasone should be avoided because they increase the mobilisation of calcium from bones and have been reported to aggravate osteolytic lesions[105].

Effect on neurological symptoms from cerebral metastases
Corticosteroids often have a dramatically beneficial effect on the neurological symptoms from brain metastases[18]. Improvement is not restricted to metastases from breast cancer and is believed to result from the resorption of oedematous and inflammatory reaction in and around the tumour deposit. The improvement in the neurological picture is often rapid and dramatic. Changes sometimes appear within hours, but more often gradually develop over a period of days. Amelioration bears not only on manifestations of intracranial hypertension but also on focal neurological disorders. In a series of 22 patients, remarkable temporary improvement was seen in 14 patients[18]. The recommended dosage in such an emergency situation is 60–100 mg of prednisolone daily, which is then gradually tapered to 60 mg daily as control of the symptoms is achieved, and to 30 mg when the patient is ambulatory. Dexamethasone is effective in doses 6 times smaller. Discontinuance of therapy usually results in rapid reversal of the neurological picture. In addition, when the disease progresses, larger doses of corticoids are required to maintain a satisfactory control.

Because endocrine therapy in general usually fails to induce regression of cerebral metastases, palliative treatment with corticosteroids is often complemented with cytotoxic chemotherapy which, in contrast, is often effective[106].

MODE OF ACTION OF CORTICOSTEROIDS IN BREAST CANCER
It is likely, although not proven, that true objective remissions, namely tumour regression, induced by corticosteroid administration result from the suppression of ACTH secretion and consequently of adrenal cortical steroid secretion. The adrenal-originated steroids which maintain breast cancer growth are believed to be the oestrogens. The adrenal cortex of man is known to produce oestrogenic steroids, probably mostly by secretion of androgens which are peripherally transformed into oestrogens, mainly in the fatty tissue[107].

An important question is whether post-menopausal ovaries still contribute to the endogenous production of oestrogens. Assuming that they still do so, various authors subjected their post-menopausal patients to ovarian ablation before initiating a corticosteroid suppressive therapy[102–104] (see above). However, there is little evidence in favour of this view. The experimental data of Nissen–Meyer and Sander[108] purporting to provide such evidence by measuring the 24-h urinary excretion of oestrone before and after ovarian ablation in postmenopausal women are in fact inconclusive because the small differences observed were not statistically significant. Barlow et al.[109] presented evidence to the contrary by showing that surgical oöphorectomy did not modify the oestradiol production rate, as measured by an isotopic dilution technique, in postmenopausal women. Again, their data are inconclusive because the measurements were done under ACTH stimulation, which could have concealed a small ACTH-unaffected contribution of the ovaries in this non-physiological situation. It is our opinion that the question remains unsettled. Furthermore, the suppressibility of adrenal-originated oestrogens by tolerable doses of corticosteroids in advanced breast cancer patients has not yet been established and may prove difficult[110]. The recent advent of sensitive radioimmunoassay methods for measuring blood oestrogens will probably make it possible to answer these two questions in the near future.

Independently of objective remissions, corticosteroids often induce marked clinical improvement. This probably results from the anti-inflammatory properties of corticosteroids. Decrease in inflammatory reactions and oedema around tumour infiltrations probably accounts for such effects as alleviation of bone or liver pain, decrease in lymphoedema and serous effusions, improvement of myelophtisic anaemia, and disappearance of neurological symptoms resulting from brain metastases. Control of hypercalcaemia also involves a specific effect on calcium metabolism (see above).

DOSAGE AND SIDE-EFFECTS

It appears from the foregoing discussion that the minimum dose of prednisolone effecting objective remission is about 10 mg three times daily. At that dosage level, side-effects are usually mild, consisting of some puffiness of the face and ankle as well as slight increase in hirsuties in most patients, and only occasionally mild dyspepsia or euphoria; hypomania was observed in only one of 80 patients treated[96]. Subjective improvement of the type described above, with only "mixed" objective response, is obtained with 5 mg prednisolone, 3 times daily, or 1 mg dexamethasone, 3 times daily. These doses are associated with very few side-effects.

High dosage levels of 50–100 mg prednisolone, or 10–30 mg dexamethasone daily, which are recommended in specific emergency situations, produce considerable side-effects when given for more than a few weeks[98]. These include weight gain, moon faces, hirsutism and abnormal fat deposition. In a series of 45 patients, the following specific complications were observed: sleeplessness and nervousness in 2 cases; psychotic symptoms in 2 cases; induction or aggravation of pre-existing diabetes in many patients; gastric or duodenal ulcers in 5 patients (2 of them had gastrointestinal bleeding, another one had a perforation as the first sign of an ulcer); quadriceps weakness in many cases; infections, acne and oedema also occurred.

If corticosteroids have been used for long periods, they should be tapered off slowly, over 1–2 weeks in order to avoid acute adrenal insufficiency. In addition, a course of slow acting ACTH (80 units tapered on successive days to 20 units) has been recommended[47].

Table 5.8 INCIDENCE OF OBJECTIVE REMISSIONS FROM OESTROGEN ANTAGONISTS TAMOXIFEN AND NAFOXIDINE

Author	Compound	Dosage (mg/day orally)	Remissions No.*	%
Cole et al.[19]	Tamoxifen	10–20	10/46	22
Ward[119]	Tamoxifen	20–40	26/68	38†
E.O.R.T.C. Breast Cancer Group[20]	Nafoxidine	180	8/23	35
Engelsman et al.[124]	Nafoxidine	180	7/30	23
Heuson et al.[118]‡	Nafoxidine	180	20/61	33 ⎫ n.s.
	Ethinyl oestradiol	3	13/59	22 ⎭

* Objective remissions/No. patients treated

† Incidence of "definite response" (reduction in size to between 50 and zero %), judged only on primary breast cancer, recurrence on chest wall or soft tissue metastases, without taking into account distant metastases; an additional 18% incidence of "partial responses" was reported

‡ Randomised comparative trial; preliminary results, not reviewed as yet

Oestrogen antagonists

EXPERIMENTAL BASIS AND HISTORICAL BACKGROUND

Oestrogen antagonists were tested as a treatment of advanced breast cancer independently by Cole et al.[19] and by the E.O.R.T.C. Breast Cancer Group[20]. The compounds used were Tamoxifen (ICI 46474 = trans isomer of 1 (p-β-dimethylaminoethoxy-phenyl)-1,2-diphenylbut-1-ene) and Nafoxidine hydrochloride (U11,100A = 1-{2-[p-(3,4-dihydro-6-methoxy-2-phenyl-1-naphtyl)phenoxy]-ethyl}-pyrrolidine hydrochloride) respectively.

Both compounds inhibit the oestrogen-induced increase in uterine weight in oöphorectomised or immature rats[111,112]. They also have a weak oestrogenic activity in rats when given in large doses as measured by their uterotrophic effect[111,112]. They prevent oestradiol retention in the uterus, both in vivo[113] and in vitro[114]. They seem to exert this effect by competitively inhibiting the binding of oestradiol to its specific uterine receptors[115]. Nafoxidine also prevents oestradiol retention in vitro in the DMBA-induced, hormone-dependent rat mammary carcinoma[114] and in human breast cancers[57]. Moreover, it has anti-tumour effects on the rat mammary carcinoma: it prevents tumour induction[116] and inhibits tumour growth[116,117]. These interesting properties led to a trial of Tamoxifen and Nafoxidine in breast cancer.

INCIDENCE OF OBJECTIVE REMISSIONS

The incidence of objective remissions induced by oestrogen antagonists is shown in Table 5.8. The remission rates were comparable to those observed with other effective hormones. It was slightly higher with Nafoxidine than with ethinyl oestradiol in a randomised comparative trial, although the difference was not statistically significant[118].

SIDE-EFFECTS

Tamoxifen displayed remarkably little side-effects at the dosages used[19,119]. Hot flushes were reported to have occurred in 12–15% and mild gastrointestinal intolerance in 13%. Vaginal bleeding was observed in only 1 case. Hypercalcaemia was not recorded. Mild transient thrombocytopenia, with counts between 50 000 and 100 000 per mm³, occurred in about 8% of cases but subsided without discontinuation of therapy.

Nafoxidine-induced marked photosensitivity occured in 13 of 26 patients. It consisted of skin erythema on direct or even indirect exposure to sunlight during summer, without resulting burn or tan. In the initial report[20], alopecia occurred in one patient and mild ichthyosis of the skin in another. However, further experience[118] disclosed a much higher rate of these complications, especially in very old women. Impressive ichthyosis was sometimes observed with scaling, redness and atrophy of skin. The face was spared. Except for cosmetic and practical inconveniences, this complication was symptomless. Pruritis occasionally occurred as a result of a typical allergic reaction. Variable degrees of hair loss was also observed in elderly women. Hypercalcaemia developed in 1 case[20]. Photosensitivity and ichthyosis were reversible on discontinuation of therapy; however, they should be considered a significant side-effect that depreciates Nafoxidine as a first-choice drug in old women. Decreasing the dose to 30 mg daily almost entirely suppressed these side-effects in a small series of patients so treated, but the therapeutic effectiveness of the lowered dosage could not yet be assessed (unplublished).

Tamoxifen was not observed significantly to influence vaginal cytology, while Nafoxidine induced an oestrogenic pattern in 11 of 14 patients examined[20].

MODE OF ACTION
While both Tamoxifen and Nafoxidine are oestrogen antagonists, they are also weakly oestrogenic in experimental animals. Tamoxifen in doses of 10–20 mg daily failed to alter the vaginal cytology in patients but Nafoxidine at the dose of 180 mg was distinctly oestrogenic. In view of the latter observation, it is unlikely that this class of compound derives its therapeutic effectiveness in post-menopausal breast cancer patients from

their anti-oestrogenic activity. Rather, it is tempting to speculate that they bind to oestrogen receptors in breast cancer tissue and thereby produce inhibitory effects of unknown nature on the cancer cells. This hypothesis finds some support in the fact that Nafoxidine is selectively active in patients having oestrogen receptors in their cancer tissue[56].

In view of a possible role of prolactin in the control of breast cancer growth (see below), it is interesting to note that whilst oestrogens appear to stimulate prolactin secretion in breast cancer, Nafoxidine lacks this effect and may even be inhibitory[55]. The bearing of this observation is unclear.

Inhibitors of prolactin secretion

It has been conclusively shown that prolactin, besides other hormones, plays a prominent part in the maintenance of growth of the DMBA-induced rat mammary carcinoma, which is often regarded as an interesting experimental model for human breast cancer[120]. It was also found that 2-Br-α-ergocryptine (CB 154), an ergot alkaloid which selectively inhibits the release of pituitary prolactin in the rat[116,121], also inhibits tumour induction and growth in the DMBA-induced rat mammary tumour system[116,122].

Although a possible role of prolactin in human breast cancer remains entirely controversial[54], the foregoing observations in the rat prompted the E.O.R.T.C. Breast Cancer Group[21] to undertake a clinical trial of CB 154 in advanced breast cancer. In a series of 19 post-menopausal women, none responded to this prolactin-inhibiting alkaloid. Another inhibitor of prolactin secretion in the rat, the cyclic imide derivative CG 603, failed to achieve significant remissions in advanced breast cancer[22]. More recently, isolated cases of remissions were reported from L-dopa administration[23,123]. However, in a controlled study by the E.O.R.T.C. Breast Cancer Group[124], L-dopa failed to achieve a single case of remission in 28 patients while Nafoxidine induced objective remissions in 7 of 30 patients (23%). In order to cast light on the situation, the relative inhibitory potency of CB 154, CG 603 and L-dopa on prolactin secretion was carefully assessed in groups of post-menopausal women[125]. Each compound was administered for several weeks.

The mean 24-hour prolactin level, as determined on samples taken every 2 hours, was measured on 2 occasions and compared to the pre-treatment level. It was found that CG 603 was totally inactive, that L-dopa was weakly though significantly effective, and that CB 154 was strongly inhibitory. With the latter compound, only about 25% of the basal level remained during treatment. If prolactin were actually involved in human breast cancer, these results indicate that CB 154 would be the drug of choice among the inhibitors of prolactin secretion presently available. Its failure to induce remissions in breast cancer[21] reflects the fact either that prolactin is not involved in the mechanisms controlling growth of this tumour or that a more complete suppression of prolactin than that achieved by CB 154 is required to induce remission. Whatever the explanation is, it is clear that L-dopa is not a promising drug unless it acts in breast cancer through mechanisms other than prolactin inhibition.

Comparison of compounds and general conclusions

PALLIATIVE EFFECTS OF HORMONE ADMINISTRATION

It is apparent from this review that hormones of different classes induce objective and valuable remissions in cases of inoperable, recurrent or advanced breast cancer. The incidence of remission lies between 20 and 30% and their median duration between 8 and 12 months. Objective remissions result in substantial clinical improvement. Some hormones like androgens and corticosteroids add subjective favourable effects, though often short-lived, through mechanisms unrelated to hormone dependence of breast cancer. Slow-growing tumours, namely those with a long free interval, are associated with a higher incidence of remission; the same holds true for patients who are more than 5 years post-menopausal as compared to those who are less. Likewise, soft tissue lesions respond better than osseous or visceral deposits, and patients suffering from soft tissue lesions only have a more favourable outlook than those having osseous or visceral metastases. Finally, a most important observation is that hormone remitters have an impressively longer survival than non-remitters, either because they belong to a privileged subgroup of patients who are "recognised" by their ability to respond, or because hormonally-induced remissions actually prolong survival, or even possibly through operation of both mechanisms. Another important, though most frustrating observation is that hormone administration, just as hormone deprivation by ablative procedures never achieves cure of breast cancer.

HORMONE ADMINISTRATION vs. ABLATIVE PROCEDURES

The first question is whether ablative procedures are more effective than hormone administration in the control of breast cancer. In *pre-menopausal* women, the remission rate from androgen administration is about 20%[15] while that obtained from surgical oöphorectomy was 29.7%[126] and 24.5%[127] respectively in 2 large series using strict criteria of objective remission. This suggests a definite advantage of oöphorectomy over hormone administration. However, it should be recognised that these figures relate to different series of patients and are not strictly comparable. To our knowledge, a randomised comparative study of androgens and surgical oöphorectomy has not been carried out. In *post-menopausal* women, it is often maintained that major ablative procedures are more effective than hormone administration. In order to investigate this point, Dao and Tan[128] conducted a randomised trial comparing androgen administration (fluoxymesterone, 20 mg/day, orally) and adrenalectomy. The respective incidences of objective remissions were 9 of 46 and 23 of 49, thus strongly favouring adrenalectomy. This isolated study deserves confirmation with other androgenic, as well as with oestrogenic compounds in order unequivocally to establish the superiority of adrenalectomy over hormone administration.

OESTROGENS vs. ANDROGENS

Relative effectiveness
A second question relates to the relative efficacy of the various hormones used in the therapy of breast cancer. In this regard, little is known in *pre-menopausal* women. Oöphorectomy is usually performed as the treatment of choice before resorting to

Table 5.9 INCIDENCE OF OBJECTIVE REMISSIONS FROM ANDROGENS AND OESTROGENS*

Interval since menopause	Androgen Remissions†	%	Oestrogen Remissions†	%	P
Post-menopausal					
0 through 8 yr	23/215	16.3	20/74	27%	<0.06
9 or more yr	46/166	27.7	89/236	37.7%	<0.05
Unknown interval	11/39	28.2	25/47	53.2%	

* A.M.A. Council on Drugs[15]
† Objective remissions/No. patients treated

Table 5.10 AVERAGE SURVIVAL OF PATIENTS ACCORDING TO TREATMENT*

Response to treatment	Androgen Patients No.	Average Mo.	Oestrogen Patients No.	Average Mo.	P
All patients	423	11.4	243	16.5	<0.001
No regression	345	9.7	156	10.4	...
Regression	78	19.1	87	27.3	<0.005

* A.M.A. Council on Drugs[15]

Table 5.11 RANDOMISED COMPARATIVE TRIALS OF ANDROGEN AND OESTROGEN

Author	Testosterone propionate Remission*	%	Diethylstilboestrol Remission*	%	P
Cooperative Breast					
Cancer Group[13]†	18/184	9.7	28/185	15.1	...
Kennedy[129]	6/59	10.1	16/55	29.1	0.022

* Objective remissions/No. patients treated
† Recalculated from Table 5.1 of this publication, after subtraction of cases contributed to by Kennedy

administrative measures. Whether androgens are more effective than oestrogens or oestrogen antagonists after oöphorectomy is still unclear. In *post-menopausal* women, some data relevant to this question are available. In the large non-randomised trial of the A.M.A. Council on Drugs[15], oestrogens and androgens were compared as to incidence of objective remissions (Table 5.9) as well as to effect on survival (Table 5.10). Both comparisons show considerable advantage in favour of oestrogen therapy. However, it should be stressed again that the treatment groups were not randomised and cannot be considered strictly comparable. Additional information can be derived from two randomised trials conducted respectively by the Cooperative Breast Cancer Group[13] and by Kennedy[129]. The results are given in Table 5.11. In both series, the incidence of remission was higher with oestrogen than with androgen therapy. In the second series, the difference was statistically significant. However, in contrast to the study of the A.M.A. Council on Drugs, the median durations of remission were not significantly different in the two treatment groups, nor was the median duration of survival in the responders to these treatments.

These three studies concur to indicate that oestrogen therapy may be more effective than androgen therapy in terms of rate of remission but only one of them suggests that oestrogen remitters have a longer survival than responders to androgen treatment.

Attempts have been made to increase the therapeutic effectiveness of hormones by combining oestrogen and androgen administration. It was found that the combination was no more effective than either hormone alone and that untoward reactions were more severe[130,131].

Comparative evaluation of side-effects
Besides therapeutic effectiveness, quality of remission is of major concern especially in patients enjoying long remissions. Side-effects of hormones must therefore be taken into careful consideration. The most frequent and troublesome adverse reaction to oestrogens is digestive intolerance. However, it occurs at the beginning of administration and usually subsides later.

Discontinuance of therapy is rarely necessary. This complication is therefore of little import on the long term. On the other hand, the major side-effects of androgens result from their virilising properties. Hoarseness, hirsutism, alopecia, acne and excessive libido are indeed most undesirable consequences which gradually build up during the course of therapy and eventually belittle the benefit gained from the remission. The feeling of well-being which is frequently obtained at the beginning of treatment is undoubtedly valuable, but often rather short-lived. It is our opinion that in patients who, according to the various predictive factors now available, both clinical and biological (see last section), are probable responders, oestrogen administration should be preferred to androgen therapy. The latter is of greater value in debilitated, very ill patients. Experience may show that compounds with lesser virilising activity, such as 2α-methyl-dihydrotestosterone propionate (Dromostanolone, Masteril) or even better Δ1-testololactone, are very valuable drugs, provided it is demonstrated that their activity is as great as that of oestrogens.

Both oestrogens and androgens may induce hypercalcaemia in patients with osseous metastases; both produce salt and water retention that can usually be controlled by appropriate measures. Uterine bleeding caused by oestrogens is only rarely a serious complication.

THE SPECIAL CASE OF CORTICOSTEROIDS
Corticosteroids occupy a unique situation in the hormonal management of breast cancer. For reasons that remain unclear, "medical adrenalectomy" proved disappointing. The incidence of objective remissions seems less than with surgical adrenalectomy or administration of sex hormones. Nevertheless, corticosteroids are of very great value in certain specific situations, probably by virtue of their anti-inflammatory properties. Subjective effects, sometimes adding to the objective benefit, may lead to major clinical improvement.

INVESTIGATIONAL COMPOUNDS
Orally-active progestogens are undoubtedly capable of producing objective remissions. The precise incidence of favourable responses is difficult to assess, owing to the smallness of the

available series. In view of its excellent tolerance, medroxy-progesterone acetate is the drug of choice in this class.

Finally, oestrogen antagonists have been recently introduced and found quite promising. Nafoxidine induces a high remission rate, that compares favourably with that obtained with oestrogens. However, at the dosage used so far, this compound produces significant skin and hair changes. Tamoxifen proved effective and remarkably devoid of serious side-effects. Both compounds certainly deserve further investigation.

Drug-induced inhibition of prolactin secretion is the subject of current investigations. However, at the time this book is written, there is no clear evidence that remissions have been induced by this mechanism, nor is there any indication that prolactin plays an appreciable part in human breast cancer.

PROSPECTS OF HORMONAL THERAPY

This review of extensive investigations on hormone therapy of breast cancer demonstrates the definite though limited usefulness of this treatment modality. Only little progress has been achieved in the field during recent years. This does not rule out the possibility, based on a better understanding of the mechanisms involved, of improving the effectiveness of hormone treatment. However, a better outlook may possibly be expected from attempt to associate cytotoxic chemotherapy and hormone therapy. The current investigative efforts should probably be made in this direction.

REFERENCES

1. Beatson, G. T. (1896). On the treatment of inoperable cases of carcinoma of the mamma. Suggestion for a new method of treatment with illustrative cases. *Lancet*, **ii**, 104

2. Adair, F. E., Treves, N., Farrow, J. H. and Scharnagel, I. M. (1945). Clinical effects of surgical and X-ray castration in mammary cancer. *J. Amer. Med. Ass.*, **128**, 161

3. Ahlbom, H. (1930). Castration by roentgen rays as an auxiliary treatment in the radiotherapy of cancer mammae at Radiumhemmet, Stockholm. *Acta Radiol.* (*Ther.*) (*Stockholm*), **11**, 614

4. Lacassagne, A. (1938). Apparition d'adénocarcinomes mammaires chez des souris mâles traitées par une substance oestrogène synthétique. *C.R. Soc. Biol.* (*Paris*), **129**, 611

5. Lacassagne, A. and Raynaud, A. (1939). Sur le mécanisme d'une action préventive de la testostérone sur le cancer mammaire de la souris. *C.R. Soc. Biol. (Paris)*, **131**, 586

6. Nathanson, I. T. and Andervont, H. B. (1939). Effect of testosterone propionate on development and growth of mammary carcinoma in female mice. *Proc. Soc. Exp. Biol. Med.*, **40**, 421

7. Badger, G. M., Elson, L. A., Haddow, A., Hewett, C. L. and Robinson, A. M. (1942). The inhibition of growth by chemical compounds. *Proc. Roy. Soc. Lond. (Biol.)*, **130**, 255

8. Loeser, A. (1939). Male hormone in the treatment of cancer of the breast. *Acta Unio. Int. Contra. Cancro.*, **4**, 375

9. Ulrich, P. (1939). Testostérone (hormone mâle) et son rôle possible dans le traitement de certains cancers du sein. *Acta Unio. Int. Contra. Cancro.*, **4**, 377

10. Ellis, F. and others (1944). Stilboestrol for advanced breast cancer. *Brit. Med. J.*, **ii**, 20

11. Ellis, F. and others (1944). Discussion on advanced cases of carcinoma of the breast treated by stilboestrol. *Proc. Roy. Soc. Med.*, **37**, 731

12. Haddow, A., Watkinson, J. M., Paterson, E. and Koller, P. C. (1944). Influence of synthetic oestrogen upon advanced malignant disease. *Brit. Med. J.*, **ii**, 393

13. Cooperative Breast Cancer Group: Progress report (1964). Results of studies of the Cooperative Breast Cancer Group 1961–1963. *Cancer Chemother. Rep.*, **41 (suppl. 1)**, 1

14. Cooperative Breast Cancer Group (1964). Testosterone propionate therapy in breast cancer. *J. Amer. Med. Ass.*, **188**, 1069

15. Council on Drugs (1960). Androgens and estrogens in the treatment of disseminated mammary carcinoma. Retrospective study of nine hundred forty-four patients. Report to the Council. *J. Amer. Med. Ass.*, **172**, 1271

16. Kennedy, B. J. and Nathanson, I. T. (1953). Effects of intensive sex steroid hormone therapy in advanced breast cancer, report to the Council on Pharmacy and Chemistry. *J. Amer. Med. Ass.*, **152**, 1135

17. Taylor, S. G. III, Slaughter, D. P., Smejkal, W., Fowler, E. F. and Preston, F. W. (1948). The effect of sex hormones on advanced carcinoma of breast. *Cancer*, **1**, 604

18. Kofman, S., Garvin, J. S., Nagamani, D. and Taylor, S. G. III (1957). Treatment of cerebral metastases from breast carcinoma with prednisolone. *J. Amer. Med. Ass.*, **163**, 1473

19. Cole, M. P., Jones, C. T. A. and Todd, I. D. H. (1971). A new anti-oestrogenic agent in late breast cancer. An early clinical appraisal of ICI 46474. *Brit. J. Cancer*, **25**, 270

20. E.O.R.T.C. Breast Cancer Group (1972). Clinical trial of Nafoxidine, an oestrogen antagonist in advanced breast cancer. *Eur. J. Cancer*, **8**, 387

21. E.O.R.T.C. Breast Cancer Group (1972). Clinical trial of 2-Br-α-ergocryptine (CB 154) in advanced breast cancer. *Eur. J. Cancer*, **8**, 155

22. E.O.R.T.C. Breast Cancer Group (1972). Clinical trial of the cyclic imide 1-(morpholinomethyl)-4-phtalimido-piperidindione-2,6 (CG 603) in advanced breast cancer. *Eur. J. Cancer*, **8**, 157

23. Murray, R. M. L., Mozzaffarian, G. and Pearson, O. H. (1972). Prolactin levels with L-dopa treatment in metastatic breast carcinoma. *Prolactin and Carcinogenesis*.

Proceedings of the Fourth Tenovus Workshop, p. 158, (Edited by A. R. Boyns and K. Griffiths). Alpha Omega Alpha Publishing, Cardiff

24. Prudente, A. (1945). Postoperative prophylaxis of recurrent mammary cancer with testosterone propionate. *Surg. Gynecol. Obstet.*, **80**, 575

25. Cooperative Breast Cancer Group: Progress report (1961). Results of studies by the Cooperative Breast Cancer Group, 1956–1960. *Cancer Chemother. Rep.*, **11**, 109

26. G.E.C.A. (1967). Protocole pour les essais cliniques de traitement des cancers mammaires humains en phase avancée. *Eur. J. Cancer*, **2**, 201

27. Haddow, A. (1935). Influence of certain polycyclic hydrocarbons on the growth of the Jensen rat sarcoma. *Nature (Lond.)*, **136**, 868

28. Cook, J. W., Dodds, E. C., Hewett, C. L. and Lawson, W. (1934). Oestrogenic activity of some condensed-ring compounds in relation to their other biological activities. *Proc. Roy. Soc. Lond. (Biol.)*, **114**, 272

29. Haddow, A. and Robinson, A. M. (1937). Influence of various polycyclic hydrocarbons on growth rate of transplantable tumours. *Proc. Roy. Soc. Lond. (Biol.)*, **122**, 442

30. Noble, R. L. (1939). Effects of continuous oral administration of aqueous diethylstilboestrol solutions to rats. *J. Endocrinol.*, **1**, 128

31. Zondek, B. (1936). Impairment of anterior pituitary functions by follicular hormone. *Lancet*, **ii**, 842

32. Gardner, W. U. and De Vita, J. (1940). Malignant and non-malignant uterine and vaginal lesions in mice receiving estrogens, and estrogens and androgens simultaneously. *Yale J. Biol. Med.*, **13**, 213

33. Hooker, C. W., Gardner, W. U. and Pfeiffer, C. A. (1940). Testicular tumors in mice receiving estrogens. *J. Amer. Med. Ass.*, **115**, 443

34. Gardner, W. U. (1941). Inhibition of mammary growth by large amounts of estrogen. *Endocrinology*, **28**, 53

35. Huggins, C. and Hodges, C. V. (1941). Studies of prostatic cancer: I. The effect of castration, of estrogen and of androgen injection on serum phosphatases in metastatic carcinoma of the prostate. *Cancer Res.*, **1**, 292

36. Biden, W. M. (1943). Stilboestrol for breast tumour. *Brit. Med. J.*, **ii**, 57

37. Nathanson, I. T. (1952). Clinical investigative experience with steroid hormones in breast cancer. *Cancer*, **5**, 754

38. Nathanson, I. T. and Kelley, R. M. (1952). Hormonal treatment of cancer. *N. Engl. J. Med.*, **246**, 135

39. Stoll, B. A. (1950). Hormone therapy in relation to radiotherapy in the treatment of advanced carcinoma of the breast. *Proc. Roy. Soc. Med.*, **43**, 875

40. Pearson, O. H., West, C. D., Hollander, V. P. and Treves, N. E. (1954). Evaluation of endocrine therapy for advanced breast cancer. *J. Amer. Med. Ass.*, **154**, 234

41. Kennedy, B. J. (1962). Massive estrogen administration in premenopausal women with metastatic breast cancer. *Cancer*, **15**, 641

42. Nemoto, T. and Dao, T. L. (1966). Significance of liver metastases in women with disseminated breast cancer undergoing endocrine ablative surgery. *Cancer*, **19**, 421

43. Huseby, R. A. (1958). The use of estrogen in the treatment of advanced breast cancer. *Breast Cancer. The Second Biennial Louisiana Cancer Conference*, p. 206. (Edited by A. Segaloff), The C. V. Mosby Company, St-Louis

44. Escher, G. C. Clinical improvement of inoperable breast carcinoma under steroid treatment. In *Proc. of the 1st conference on steroid hormones and mammary carcinoma.* April 1949, pp. 92–99. Therapeutic trials Committee, Council on Pharmac. and Chemistry of the American Medical Association

45. Baker, L. H. and Vaitkevicius, V. K. (1972). Reevaluation of rebound regression in disseminated carcinoma of the breast. *Cancer*, **29**, 1268

46. Kaufman, R. J. and Escher, G. C. (1961). Rebound regression in advanced mammary carcinoma. *Surg. Gynecol. Obstet.*, **113**, 635

47. Stoll, B. A. (1969). *Hormonal Management in Breast Cancer.* Pitman Med. Publishing Cy. Ltd.

48. Keating, J. L., Yonemoto, R. H. and Byron, R. L. (1968). Cytotoxic drug and hormone therapy after adrenalectomy for advanced breast cancer. *Surg. Gynecol. Obstet.*, **127**, 538

49. Pearson, O. H. and Ray, B. S. (1959). Results of hypophysectomy in the treatment of metastatic mammary carcinoma. *Cancer*, **12**, 85

50. Talley, R. W., Brennan, M. J., Vaitkevicius, V. K., San Diego, E. L., Reed, M. L. and Leighton, G. A. (1964). Comparison of 6α-methyl-9α-fluoro-17-acetoxy-21-deoxyprednisolone with fluoxymesterone and methyl prednisolone in treatment of metastatic breast cancer. *Cancer*, **17**, 1063

51. Kim, U. (1965). Pituitary function and hormonal therapy of experimental breast cancer. *Cancer Res.*, **25**, 1146

52. Lerner, L. J. and Hilf, R. (1967). Biological activities of steroids and their relationship to breast cancer therapy. *Current Concepts in Breast Cancer*, p. 80. (Edited by A. Segaloff, K. K. Meyer and S. Debakey) The Williams and Wilkins Company, Baltimore

53. Meites, J. and Nicoll, C. S. (1966). Adenohypophysis: prolactin. *Annu. Rev. Physiol.*, **28**, 57

54. Heuson, J. C. (1974). The role of prolactin inhibition in [the] treatment [of breast cancer]. *Mammary Cancer and Neuroendocrine Therapy.* p. 349 (Edited by B. Stoll). Butterworth, London.

55. L'Hermite, M., Heuson, J. C., Rozencweig, M. and Robyn, Cl. (1974). Breast cancer regression under oestrogen therapy. *Brit. Med. J.*, **1**, 390.

56. Engelsman, E., Persijn, J. P., Korsten, C. B. and Cleton, F. J. (1973). Oestrogen receptor in human breast cancer tissue and response to endocrine therapy. *Brit. Med. J.*, **2**, 750

57. Jensen, E. V., Block, G. E., Smith, S., Kyser, K. and DeSombre, E. R. (1971). Estrogen receptors and hormone dependency. *Estrogen Target Tissue and Neoplasia.* (Edited by T. L. Dao). The University of Chicago Press, Chicago and London

58. Maass, H., Engel, B., Hohmeister, H., Lehmann, F. and Trams, G. (1972). Estrogen receptors in human breast cancer tissue. *Am. J. Obstet. Gynecol.*, **113**, 377

59. Emerson, W. J., Kennedy, B. J., Graham, J. N. and Nathanson, I. T. (1953). Pathology of primary and recurrent carcinoma of the human breast after administration of steroid hormones. *Cancer*, **6**, 641

60. Hall, T. C., Dederick, M. M. and Nevinny, H. B. (1963). Prognostic value of hormonally induced hypercalcemia in breast cancer. *Cancer Chemother. Rep.*, **30**, 21

61. Beckett, V. L. (1969). Hypercalcemia associated with estrogen administration in patients with breast carcinoma. *Cancer*, **24**, 610

62. Galasko, C. S. B. and Burn, I. (1971). Hypercalcemia in patients with advanced mammary cancer. *Brit. Med. J.*, **3**, 573

63. Veterans Administration Co-operative Urological Research Group (1967). Treatment and survival of patients with cancer of the prostate. *Surg. Gynecol. Obstet.*, **124**, 1011

64. Fels, E. (1944). Treatment of breast cancer with testosterone propionate. *J. Clin. Endocrinol. Metab.*, **4**, 121

65. Farrow, J. H. and Woodard, H. O. (1942). The influence of androgenic and estrogenic substances on serum calcium in cases of skeletal metastases from mammary cancer. *J. Amer. Med. Ass.*, **18**, 339

66. Adair, F. E. and Herrmann, J. B. (1946). Use of testosterone propionate in treatment of advanced carcinoma of breast. *Ann. Surg.*, **123**, 1023

67. de Lorimier, A. A., Gordan, G. S., Lowe, R. C. and Carbone, J. V. (1965). Methyltestosterone, related steroids and liver function. *Arch. Intern. Med.*, **116**, 289

68. Beckett, V. L. and Brennan, M. J. (1959). Treatment of advanced breast cancer with fluoxymesterone (Halotestin). *Surg. Gynecol. Obstet.*, **109**, 235

69. Segaloff, A., Weeth, J. B., Rongone, E. L., Murison, P. J. and Bowers, C. Y. (1960). Hormonal therapy in cancer of the breast. XVI. The effect of Δ1-testololactone on clinical course and hormonal excretion. *Cancer*, **13**, 1017

70. Groupe Européen du Cancer du Sein (1962). Le traitement hormonal du cancer du sein. *Rev. Eur. Etud. Clin. Biol.*, **7**, 1067

71. Goldenberg, I. S., Waters, M. N., Ravdin, R. S., Ansfield, F. J. and Segaloff, A. (1973). Androgenic therapy for advanced breast cancer in women. *J. Amer. Med. Ass.*, **223**, 1267

72. Gordan, G. S., Halden, A., Horn, Y., Fuery, J. J., Parsons, R. J. and Walter, R. M. (1973). Calusterone (7β,17α-dimethyltestosterone) as primary and secondary therapy of advanced breast cancer. *Oncology*, **28**, 138

73. Gordon, D., Horwitt, B. N., Segaloff, A., Murison, P. J. and Schlosser, J. V. (1952). Hormonal therapy in cancer of the breast. III. Effect of progesterone on clinical course and hormonal excretion. *Cancer*, **5**, 275

74. Taylor, S. G., III, and Morris, R. S., Jr. (1951). Hormones in breast metastasis therapy. *Med. Clin. North. Am.*, **35**, 51

75. Crowley, L. G. and Macdonald, I. (1962). Clinical trial of Delalutin in the treatment of advanced mammary carcinoma in postmenopausal women. *Cancer*, **15**, 1218

76. Jones, V., Joslin, C. A. F., Jones, R. E., Davies, D. K. L., Roberts, M. M., Gleave, E. N., Campbell, H., Forrest, A. P. M. (1971). Progestogens and advanced breast cancer. *Lancet*, **i**, 1049

77. Crowley, L. G. and Macdonald, I. (1965). Delalutin and estrogens for the treatment of advanced mammary carcinoma in the postmenopausal woman. *Cancer*, **18**, 436

78. Ahmann, D. L., Hahn, R. G. and Bisel, H. F. (1972). Disseminated breast cancer: evaluation of hormonal therapy utilizing stilboestrol and Medrogestone (Ay-62022) singly and in combination. *Cancer*, **30**, 651

79. Berndt, G. und Stender, H. St. (1970). Die Östrogen-Gestagen-Kombinations-behandlung des metastasierenden Mammakarzinoms mit SH 834. *Dtsch. Med. Wochenschr.*, **48**, 2399

80. Landau, R. L., Ehrlich, E. N. and Huggins, C. (1962). Estradiol benzoate and progesterone in advanced human-breast cancer. *J. Amer. Med. Ass.*, **182**, 632

81. Stoll, B. A. (1967). Effect of Lyndiol, an oral contraceptive, on breast cancer. *Brit. Med. J.*, **1**, 150

82. Talley, R. W., O'Bryan, R. M., Burrows, J. H. and San Diego, E. L. (1970). Comparison of Δ1-Testololactone and an estrogen progestin combination in the treatment of metastatic breast cancer. *Cancer Chemother. Rep.*, **54**, 249

83. Goldenberg, I. S. and Hayes, M. A. (1959). Hormonal therapy of metastatic female breast cancer. I. 9α-Fluoro-11-keto-progesterone. *Cancer*, **12**, 738

84. Jonsson, U., Colsky, J., Lessner, H. E., Roath, O. S., Alper, R. G. and Jones, R., Jr. (1959). Clinical and pharmacological observations of the effects of 9-α-bromo-11-β-ketoprogesterone in patients with carcinoma of the breast. *Cancer*, **12**, 509

85. Gorins, A. and Netter, A. (1969). L'apport des norstéroïdes dans le traitement des cancers du sein en phase avancée. *Presse Med.*, **77**, 817

86. Briggs, M. H., Caldwell, A. D. S. and Pitchford, A. G. (1967). The treatment of breast cancer by progestogens. *Hosp. Med.*, **1**, 63

87. Muggia, F. M., Cassileth, P. A., Ochoa, M., Flatow, F. A., Gellhorn, A. and Hyman, G. A. (1968). Treatment of breast cancer with medroxyprogesterone acetate. *Ann. Intern. Med.*, **68**, 3

88. Stoll, B. A. (1967). Progestin therapy of breast cancer: comparison of agents. *Brit. Med. J.*, **3**, 338

89. Kaufman, R. J., Rothschild, E. O., Escher, G. C. and Myers, W. P. L. (1964). Hypercalcemia in mammary carcinoma following the administration of a progestational agent. *J. Clin. Endocrinol. Metab.*, **24**, 1235

90. Stoll, B. A. (1966). Therapy by progestational agents in advanced breast cancer. *Med. J. Aust.*, **1**, 331

91. Volk, H., Escher, G. C., Huseby, R. A., Tyler, F. H. and Cheda, J. (1960). Hormonal therapy in carcinoma of the breast: I. Effect of oral progesterone on clinical course and metabolism of nitrogen and selected electrolytes and steroids. *Cancer*, **13**, 757

92. Carter, S. K. (1972). Single and combination nonhormonal chemotherapy in breast cancer. *Cancer*, **30**, 1543

93. Segaloff, A., Carabasi, R., Horwitt, B. N., Schlosser, J. V. and Murison, P. J. (1954). Hormonal therapy of cancer of the breast. VI. Effect of ACTH and cortisone on clinical course and hormonal excretion. *Cancer*, **7**, 331

94. Dao, T. L., Tan, E. and Brooks, V. (1961). A comparative evaluation of adrenalectomy and cortisone in the treatment of advanced mammary carcinoma. *Cancer*, **14**, 1259

95. Van Gilse, H. A. (1962). Long-term treatment with corticosteroids of patients with metastatic breast cancer. *Cancer Chemother. Rep.*, **16**, 293

96. Stoll, B. A. (1963). Corticosteroids in therapy of advanced mammary cancer. *Brit. Med. J.*, **2**, 210

97. Firat, D. and Olshin, S. (1968). Treatment of metastatic carcinoma of the female breast with combinations of hormones and other chemotherapy. *Cancer Chemother. Rep.*, **52**, 743

98. Kofman, S., Nagamani, D., Buenger, R. and Taylor, S. G., III (1958). The use of prednisolone in the treatment of disseminated breast carcinoma. *Cancer*, **11**, 226

99. Lemon, H. M. (1957). Cortisone-thyroid therapy of metastatic mammary cancer. *Ann. Intern. Med.*, **46**, 457

100. Lemon, H. M. (1959). Prednisone therapy of advanced mammary cancer. *Cancer*, **12**, 93

101. Gardner, B., Thomas, A. N. and Gordan, G. S. (1962). Antitumor efficacy of prednisone and sodium liothyronine in advanced breast cancer. *Cancer*, **15**, 334

102. Brinkley, D. M. and Kingsley Pillers, E. (1960). Treatment of advanced carcinoma of the breast by bilateral oophorectomy and prednisone. *Lancet*, **i**, 123

103. Forrest, A. P. M., Stewart, H. J., Benson, E. A., Ker, H., Jones, V., Kunkler, P. B. and Campbell, H. (1968). Controlled studies in advanced breast cancer. *Prognostic Factors in Breast Cancer*, p. 186. (Edited by A. P. M. Forrest and P. B. Kunkler). Edinburgh and London: Livingstone

104. Nissen-Meyer, R. and Vogt, J. H. (1959). Cortisone treatment of metastatic breast cancer. *Acta Unio. Int. Contra. Cancro.*, **15**, 1140

105. Stoll, B. A. (1960). Dexamethasone in advanced breast cancer. *Cancer*, **13**, 1074

106. Hildebrand, J., Brihaye, J., Wagenknecht, L., Michel, J. and Kenis, Y. (1973). Combination chemotherapy with 1-(2-chloroethyl-3-cyclohexyl-1-nitrosourea) (CCNU), vincristine and methotrexate in primary and metastatic brain tumors. A preliminary report. *Eur. J. Cancer*, **9**, 627

107. Grodin, J. M., Suteri, P. K. and MacDonald, P. C. (1973). Source of estrogen production in postmenopausal women. *J. Clin. Endocrinol. Metab.*, **36**, 207

108. Nissen-Meyer, R. and Sanner, T. (1963). The excretion of estrone, pregnanediol and pregnanetriol in breast cancer patients. *Acta Endocrinol. (Kbh)*, **44**, 334

109. Barlow, J. J., Emerson, K., Jr. and Saxena, B. N. (1969). Estradiol production after ovariectomy for carcinoma of the breast. *New Engl. J. Med.*, **280**, 633

110. Saez, J. (1971). Adrenal function in cancer: relation to the evolution. *Eur. J. Cancer*, **7**, 381

111. Duncan, G. W., Wyngarden, L. J. and Cornette, J. C. (1968). Inhibition of deciduomata development by non-steroidal antifertility agents. *J. Reprod. Fertil.* **(suppl. 4)**, 15

112. Harper, M. J. K. and Walpole, A. L. (1966). Contrasting endocrine activities of *cis* and *trans* isomers in a series of substituted triphenylethylenes. *Nature*, **212**, 87

113. Terenius, L. (1970). Two modes of interaction between oestrogen and anti-oestrogen. *Acta Endocrinol.*, **64**, 47

114. Jensen, E. V., DeSombre, E. R. and Jungblut, P. W. (1967). Estrogen receptors in hormone-responsive tissues and tumors. *International Symposium on Endogenous Factors Influencing Host-Tumor Balance*, p. 15. (Edited by R. W. Wissler, T. L. Dao and S. Wood, Jr.). The University of Chicago Press, Chicago and London

115. Steggles, A. W. and King, R. J. B. (1970). The use of protamin to study [6,7-^{3}H]-oestradiol-17β binding in rat uterus. *Biochem. J.*, **118**, 695

116. Heuson, J. C., Waelbroeck, Ch., Legros, N., Gallez, Gh., Robyn, C. and L'Hermite, M. (1971/72). Inhibition of DMBA-induced mammary carcinogenesis in the rat by 2-Br-α-ergocryptine (CB 154), an inhibitor of prolactin secretion, and by Nafoxidine (U-11, 100A), an estrogen antagonist. *Gynecol. Invest.*, **2**, 130

117. Terenius, L. (1971). Anti-oestrogens and breast cancer. *Eur. J. Cancer*, **7**, 57

118. Heuson, J. C., Engelsman, E., Blonck-Van der Wijst, D., Maas, H., Gorins, A. and Drochmans, A. (1974). Controlled trial of Nafoxidine and ethinyloestradiol

in advanced breast cancer. An E.O.R.T.C. Breast Cancer Group study. In preparation

119. Ward, H. W. C. (1973). Anti-oestrogen therapy for breast cancer: a trial of tamoxifen at two dose levels. *Brit. Med. J.*, **1**, 13

120. Pearson, O. H., Llerena, O., Llerena, L., Molina, A. and Butler, T. (1969). Prolactin-dependent rat mammary cancer: a model for man? *Trans. Ass. Am. Physicians.*, **82**, 225

121. Pasteels, J. L., Danguy, A., Frérotte, M. and Ectors, F. (1971). Inhibition de la sécrétion de prolactine par l'ergocornine et la 2-Br-α-ergocryptine: action directe sur l'hypophyse en culture. *Ann. Endocrinol.*, **32**, 188

122. Heuson, J. C., Waelbroeck-Van Gaver, C. and Legros, N. (1970). Growth inhibition of rat mammary carcinoma and endocrine changes produced by 2-Br-α-ergocryptine, a suppressor of lactation and nidation. *Eur. J. Cancer*, **6**, 353

123. Frantz, A. G., Habis, D. V., Hyman, G. A., Suh, H. K., Sassin, J. S., Zimmerman, E. A., Noel, G. L. and Kleinberg, D. L. (1973). Physiological and pharmacological factors affecting prolactin secretion, including its suppression by L-dopa in the treatment of breast cancer. *Human Prolactin*, p. 273. (Edited by J. L. Pasteels and C. Robyn). Internatl. Congress Series, no. 308. Excerpta Medica, Amsterdam. American Elsevier Publishing Cy. Inc., New York

124. Engelsman, E., Heuson, J. C., Blonk-Van der Wijst, D. and Maass, H. (1974). Controlled trial of L-dopa in advanced breast cancer. An E.O.R.T.C. Breast Cancer Group study. In preparation

125. Rozencweig, M., Heuson, J. C., Bila, S., L'Hermite, M. and Robyn, C. (1973). Effects of 2-Br-α-ergocryptine, L-dopa and cyclic imides on serum prolactin in postmenopausal women. *Eur. J. Cancer*, **9**, 657

126. Taylor, S. G. (1962). Endocrine ablation in disseminated mammary carcinoma. *Surg. Gynecol. Obstet.*, **115**, 443

127. Hall, T. C., Dederick, M. M., Nevinny, H. B. and Muench, H. (1963). Prognostic value of response of patients with breast cancer to therapeutic castration. *Cancer Chemother. Rep.*, **31**, 47

128. Dao, T. L. and Tan, E. (1962). A comparative evaluation of adrenalectomy and androgen in advanced mammary carcinoma. *Cancer Chemother. Rep.*, **16**, 309

129. Kennedy, B. J. (1965). Diethylstilbestrol versus testosterone propionate therapy in advanced breast cancer. *Surg. Gynecol. Obstet.*, **120**, 1246

130. Haines, C. R., Wallace, H. J., Nevinny, H. B. (1969). Clinical evaluation of estrogen–androgen combination in advanced breast cancer. *Am. J. Surg.*, **117**, 589

131. Kennedy, B. J. and Brown, J. H. (1965). Combined estrogenic and androgenic hormone therapy in advanced breast cancer. *Cancer*, **18**, 431

132. Stoll, B. A. (1964). Fact and fallacy in the hormonal control of breast cancer. *Med. J. Aust.*, **1**, 980

133. Stoll, B. A. (1973). Hypothesis: breast cancer regression under oestrogen therapy. *Brit. Med. J.*, **3**, 446

134. Huseby, R. A. (1954). Estrogen therapy in the management of advanced breast cancer. *Am. Surg.*, **20**, 112

135. Duncan, G. W., Lyster, S. C., Clark, J. J. and Lednicer, D. (1963). Antifertility activities of two diphenyl-dihydronaphtalene derivatives. *Proc. Soc. Exp. Biol. Med.*, **112**, 439

136. Kennedy, B. J. (1965). Hormone therapy for advanced breast cancer. *Cancer*, **18**, 1551

6

Chemotherapy of breast cancer

F. J. Ansfield

The most common malignant neoplasm afflicting women is breast cancer. Yet despite its prevalence, little progress in enhancing survival has been achieved in the last few decades.

There still remains divergence of opinion as to optimal primary treatment of this tumour, with many surgeons deviating from the classical radical mastectomy and not removing the pectoral muscles. Similarly there is no unanimity of opinion as to the utility of post-operative irradiation although it is generally agreed that this reduces the incidence of local recurrence; however the survival is not increased[1]. In a large controlled study[2] a short course of thio-TEPA used as an adjuvant following radical mastectomy also failed to enhance survival time. Finally, oöphorectomy as an adjuvant to mastectomy in pre-menopausal patients resulted in a delay in the appearance of recurrent disease but has not increased survival[3]. It is universally agreed that an urgent need exists for an effective adjuvant treatment, particularly in patients with many involved axillary nodes which bode such a dire prognosis[4].

For several decades hormonal manipulation has stood the test of time in an attempt at controlling recurrent disseminated breast cancer. Sex hormones, androgens as well as oestrogens, have produced remissions in approximately 20% of patients given adequate trial. Ablative procedures such as oöphorectomy in the pre-menopausal patient as well as adrenalectomy or hypophysectomy have afforded slightly over $\frac{1}{4}$ of the patients a useful remission. A higher regression rate from the major procedures is observed in the younger women who initially experienced an objective response to oöphorectomy and in the post-menopausal women with positive Bulbrook determinants and those with an elevated oestrogen receptor level.

In the past decade increasing use of cytotoxic drugs, particularly in patients unresponsive to hormone therapy, has come to the fore. And when the Cooperative Breast Cancer Group[5] reported that the younger post-menopausal patients, especially those with visceral metastases, were relatively unresponsive to hormones, the steroids were bypassed in them by some investigators in favour of cytotoxic drugs as the initial chemotherapy. After these were exhausted, not infrequently one or more hormonal manipulations were offered, too often with disappointing results.

Adjuvant chemotherapy

AS IMMEDIATE POST-OPERATIVE TREATMENT

Since 80% of women with 4 or more positive axillary nodes at mastectomy develop recurrence within 5 years[4] and post-operative irradiation has not increased the survival rate[1], radiotherapy was discontinued as an adjuvant 8 years ago and replaced by the prescription of 5-fluorouracil (5-FU). Not only does radiation treatment not increase survival, but it often produces morbidity consisting of varying degrees of pulmonary fibrosis, or it contributes to *lymphoedema* of the arm or to the development of a painful and persistent neuralgia over the mastectomy site. Radiotherapists usually acknowledge the fact that post-mastectomy irradiation does not increase the survival, but they plead that it does reduce the incidence of local recurrence thus affording the patients a more comfortable survival, and it has been shown that post-operative irradiation can reduce the incidence of local recurrence to less than 5%. It is true that if radiotherapy were withheld and local recurrences developed and then these were given irradiation, only 50% would have the local recurrence eradicated. Nevertheless, we believe that, in patients with any number of axillary nodes involved, the post-operative prescription of 5-FU or the 4-drug therapy described below is to be preferred. Beginning about 3 weeks after mastectomy, these high-risk patients were given 6 courses of 5-FU, each series of injections to the point of slight toxicity with 30-day intervals between courses. At the time that 31 patients who entered into this study were at risk for 5 years, 18 of them (58%)

showed no evidence of recurrence. This is a significant improvement over the historical controls where only 33% are free of disease at 5 years.

However, since almost half of the patients did develop recurrence by 5 years, 20 months ago this 5-FU adjuvant regimen was discontinued and replaced by a combination of 3 drugs given intravenously, 5-FU, 15 mg/kg weekly; methotrexate, 25 mg weekly; and vincristine, 1 mg weekly for 4 weeks, then 0.5 mg every other week; plus Megace, 160 mg daily orally. This 4-drug combination was given as an adjuvant to mastectomy in these high-risk patients with 4 or more positive axillary nodes. Of the 51 patients that received this adjuvant therapy, begun usually 2 to 3 weeks following mastectomy, no recurrences have as yet appeared. This treatment is continued for 1 year and then terminated. It is too early to predict its efficacy, with only 20 patients at risk for 18 months or more, yet in the historical controls 52% of such patients have recurrences in 18 months.

FOR LOCAL RECURRENCES
Over the past 13 years, I have used actinomycin D, 4 γ/kg/day for the first 7 days of irradiation for local recurrent breast cancer, then that same dose 3 times weekly throughout the course of radiotherapy with most satisfactory results. Failure to promote disappearance of the local recurrence was very rare except in those patients who received prior and often inadequate irradiation so that due to this earlier treatment they could not be given the full 5000 rads combined with actinomycin D, a further reason in my view for withholding immediate postoperative irradiation in such advanced cases.

It is well recognised that patients who develop local recurrence such as supraclavicular or cervical nodes, chest wall recurrences or metastasis to a vertebra can be given optimal treatment of irradiation plus actinomycin D for the soft tissue recurrence, and radiotherapy without the drug for the localised osseous metastasis. However, they are, with rare exceptions, ultimately destined to develop recurrent disseminated disease. Rather than await such a circumstance which spells doom to the patient, if all studies including a complete bone scan are negative, they are placed on the same 4-drug combination as used in the adjuvant post-mastectomy treatment but for 18 months. This is an effort to "cure" an incurable cancer patient, and the preliminary results appear promising.

Each compound individually in this 4-drug combination has proven antitumour activity against breast cancer, and none has any permanent deleterious effect on any organ system. Note that no alkylating agent is used. This was omitted by design, because if a patient had received adjuvant chemotherapy which included an alkylating agent for one year, and despite this combination of drugs the patient developed disseminated recurrent disease, then the possibility of useful palliation with hormonal manipulation as well as cytotoxic drugs is markedly reduced. Alkylating agents are termed radiomimetic, and with adequate dosage over a sufficient period of time, they permanently reduce the bone marrow potential to maintain the important white cell count and platelets so that subsequent trials with cytotoxic compounds, the antimetabolites such as 5-FU, methotrexate, etc., most antibiotic antitumour compounds as actinomycin D, adriamycin, etc., and other alkylating agents, the nitrosoamines, the mustards, etc., and even Cooper's 5-drug combination will all have to be administered in reduced, and consequently less effective dosages.

Equally disconcerting is the serious deleterious effect alkylating agents exert on subsequent hormonal treatment, both additive and ablative. Of 221 patients I treated with sex steroids under the aegis of our Cooperative Breast Cancer Group, those that had no prior chemotherapy had an 11% remission rate. However, if a previous trial with an alkylating agent had been given, sex steroids administered later produced a response in only 5.5% of the cases. 5-Fluorouracil did not appear to produce this deleterious effect. Perhaps more striking were the completely negative results of adrenalectomy and hypophysectomy, in hormonally responsive women determined primarily by virtue of previous objective responses to oöphorectomy, who received alkylating therapy at any time prior to the major ablative procedure.

Disseminated breast cancer

In the management of disseminated cancer, the menopausal age plays an important role. The pre-menopausal patient, and women up to 1 year post-menopausal, after careful baseline studies are taken including X-rays of the skull, dorso–lumbar spine, pelvis, upper end of both femora and chest, liver enzyme studies, colour photographs of all visible lesions, and caliper measurements of palpable nodules, an oöphorectomy is performed with no cytotoxic chemotherapy or hormones introduced. Then the sequence is followed as shown in Figure 6.1.

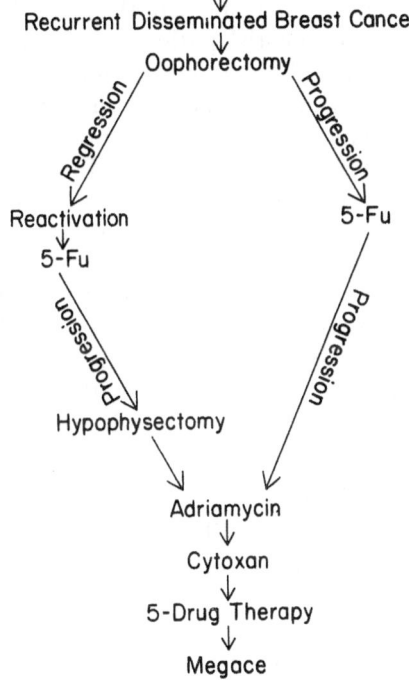

PRE-MENOPAUSAL WOMAN   MASTECTOMY

Recurrent Disseminated Breast Cancer

Oophorectomy

Regression   Progression

Reactivation   5-Fu

5-Fu

Progression   Progression

Hypophysectomy

Adriamycin

Cytoxan

5-Drug Therapy

Megace

Figure 6.1 Management of disseminated breast cancer in the premenopausal patient.

Those that respond to oöphorectomy are upon reactivation given a trial with 5-FU. This drug does not appear to interfere with subsequent responsiveness to hypophysectomy, and it is preferable to use it prior to the ablative procedure because if a loading course of 5-FU is given subsequent to hypophysectomy undue toxicity can ensue. 5-Fluorouracil is not given by single daily injection during the loading course but rather by the multiple daily dose method[6,7] which is considerably more effective with a 37% remission incidence in breast cancer as opposed to 23.1%[8] incidence when 5-FU is given by single daily injection. The dosage regimen for 5-FU given by multiple daily dose is determined by whether the patient is a good or poor risk.

POOR-RISK PATIENTS

Poor-risk patients are those who have had prior trials with an alkylating agent, osseous metastases to the pelvic bones and are over 70 years of age. A poor-risk patient is given a reduced multiple daily dose regimen of 15 mg/kg/day for 4 days followed by $\frac{1}{2}$ doses every other day until the point of slight reaction or until 11 such $\frac{1}{2}$ doses have been administered, and following termination of the course receives weekly doses of 15 mg/kg as does the good-risk patient. Additionally, some poor-risk patients are not treated with a loading course of 5-FU because of the prohibitive hazard of toxicity, and this includes patients who have had a prior adrenalectomy or hypophysectomy, extensive pelvic irradiation or extensive liver metastasis associated with jaundice. Similarly, if the oral intake is significantly curtailed or if they have a moderate to severe infection, these situations must be eliminated before 5-FU can be administered.

GOOD-RISK PATIENTS

Good-risk patients are given 5-FU at a dosage of 20 mg/kg/day for 5 days, then $\frac{1}{2}$ doses every other day to the point of slight reaction or until 11 such $\frac{1}{2}$ doses are administered at which point the course is terminated. Slight reaction includes diarrhoea to the extent of 3 fluid or semi-fluid stools a day, the appearance of an area of stomatitis on the inner surface of the lower lip covered with white pseudomembrane, a drop in the white cell count to 3500 or a significant decrease in retained oral intake. The whole doses of 20 mg/kg/day as well as the half doses are not given as a single injection, but rather they are divided into 6 equal portions, and $\frac{1}{6}$ of the dose is injected into a butterfly needle connected to a small catheter attached to a "heparin well" every 4 hours around the clock. When the good-risk patient receives 5 whole doses followed by a day of rest, then 2 half doses on alternate days and experiences no toxicity, the $\frac{1}{2}$

doses are given daily until the point of slight reaction or until 11 such doses have been administered, when the course is halted. This reduces the duration of the hospital stay. Administering the 5-FU by the multiple daily dose method renders the loading course less hazardous, because when a decision is made that the patient is eligible for a dose on morning rounds, only $\frac{1}{6}$ of the dose is given instead of the entire dose. Then if the patient develops a moderate diarrhoea or stomatitis, the course is terminated without the remaining $\frac{5}{6}$ of the dose having been given. Following termination of the loading course, the patient is sent home, returns in one week, and if the reactions have subsided and if the white blood count is adequate and stable, the patient then receives 5-FU as a single injection once weekly at a dose of 15 mg/kg/week. Whenever 5-FU is used in the obese, the ideal weight is used as an indication rather than the actual weight.

In my opinion 5-FU is the most important compound in the management of advanced breast cancer, because in the absence of progression it can be given month after month and year after year without any permanent deleterious effects on any organ system. And fortunately, it does not produce immunosuppression[9].

The question is often asked whether the loading course is essential in view of the report by Jacobs et al.[10] who stated that it is preferable to omit it and give only the weekly doses. It is my opinion that 5-FU is most effective when given to its maximum potential, and now with the advent of the multiple daily dose method of administration carrying a response rate of 37% in breast cancer with the criteria of regression including a 50% reduction in tumour size, and with the added safety factor of only $\frac{1}{6}$ of the dose given every 4 h the loading course is of prime importance.

Our Central Oncology Group is currently conducting a randomised study comparing 4 different dosage regimens of 5-FU. The first is the loading course of 12 mg/kg/day intravenously for 4 or 5 days followed by $\frac{1}{2}$ doses 4 times weekly to the point of slight reaction or until 11 such $\frac{1}{2}$ doses are given. The maximum whole dose is not to exceed 800 mg. Following the loading course, weekly doses of 15 mg/kg are given. The other regimens are Jacobs' schedule of weekly injections of 15 mg/kg with no loading course, an oral schedule of 15 mg/kg/

day for 5 or 6 days followed by 15 mg orally once weekly and a non-toxic schedule of 500 mg intravenously daily for 4 days, then 500 mg once weekly. The study is only $\frac{1}{4}$ completed, so it is too early to estimate the results by this method, but until they are available I urge a loading course, preferably by the multiple daily dose method.

Adjuvant therapy after hypophysectomy
When 5-FU fails, a hypophysectomy is then performed in patients who initially responded to oöphorectomy. Upon progression following hypophysectomy, adriamycin is administered at a dosage schedule of 0.4 mg/kg daily for 3 days, a 4 day rest period, again 3 days of therapy of 0.4 mg/kg/day and thereafter 0.4 mg/kg once weekly. In the absence of leukopenia and thrombocytopenia, the weekly dose can be elevated to 0.6 mg/kg once weekly intravenously.

PATIENTS UNSUITABLE FOR HYPOPHYSECTOMY
Patients who fail on oöphorectomy and are consequently not subjected to hypophysectomy are given a loading course of 5-FU by the multiple daily dose method followed by weekly maintenance doses, and upon progression a trial with adriamycin. Recent reports of adriamycin[11] indicated that this compound produced a remission in 75% of patients with advanced breast cancer that had had no prior chemotherapy. This dropped to only a 25% remission rate in patients who had had extensive chemotherapy, such as Cooper's 5-drug therapy[12].

Patients showing progression after adriamycin are given Cytoxan at a schedule of 400 mg/day intravenously on the first 4 days, and thereafter 150 mg daily orally after breakfast until the white cell count drops to 3000. When the count is between 3000 and 2000, 100 mg are given daily. When the count drops to under 2000, the Cytoxan is discontinued until the count recovers, and again 100 mg are administered when the count is above 2000, and so on repeatedly. Patients are cautioned to drink not less than 6 pints of fluid daily to avoid haemorrhagic cystitis. Upon progression following a trial with Cytoxan, patients are placed on 5-drug therapy in a modified Cooper's regimen as we described[13]. This consists of weekly injections of 500 mg 5-FU, 25 mg methotrexate (providing the kidney function is normal) and 1 mg vincristine for 4 weekly doses, then 0.5 mg every other week providing the deep tendon reflexes are present. In addition to the 3 drugs given intravenously, the patient receives orally 100 mg Cytoxan every morning after breakfast and prednisone 45 mg daily for the first 2 weeks, 30 mg daily for the next 2 weeks, then 15 mg daily thereafter. Any or all of the 5 drugs are reduced or withheld if toxicity ascribed to the drugs appears.

Upon failure with 5-drug therapy, if adriamycin has not been used earlier, it can be given at this time. Additionally, it has been shown that even after 5-drug therapy, Megace is valuable at a dose of 160 mg daily orally. Additive sex hormone treatment is not used in patients less than 1 year post-menopausal because the incidence of response is low.

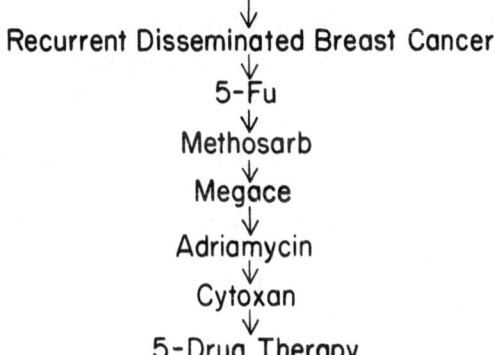

1–5 YEARS POST-MENOPAUSAL—MASTECTOMY

↓

Recurrent Disseminated Breast Cancer

↓

5-Fu

↓

Methosarb

↓

Megace

↓

Adriamycin

↓

Cytoxan

↓

5-Drug Therapy

Figure 6.2 Management of disseminated breast cancer in patients 1–5 years post-menopausal.

In the age group 1–5 years post-menopausal (Figure 6.2) patients with disseminated breast cancer are first offered a 5-FU loading course given by multiple daily dose followed by weekly doses of 15 mg/kg as described earlier. Upon failure, they are given a trial with Methosarb, very likely the most effective androgen available[14]. Usually very little virilisation occurs over the first 2–3 months, but masculinisation becomes quite evident thereafter. With progression, a trial with Megace, 160

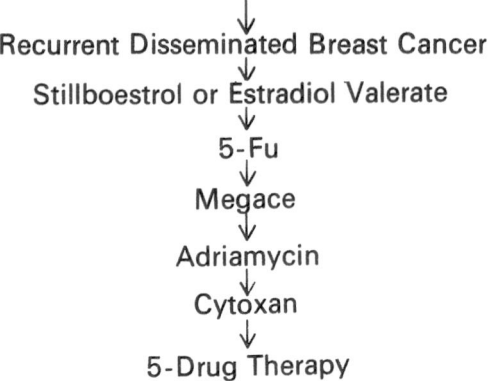

>5 YEARS POST-MENOPAUSAL—MASTECTOMY

Recurrent Disseminated Breast Cancer

Stillboestrol or Estradiol Valerate

5-Fu

Megace

Adriamycin

Cytoxan

5-Drug Therapy

Figure 6.3 Management of disseminated breast cancer in patients more than 5 years post-menopausal.

mg daily, can then be utilised. With further progression, adria-mycin is administered and finally 5-drug therapy.

Patients more than 5 years post-menopausal (Figure 6.3) are first treated with stilboestrol, starting with 5 mg at bedtime for the first 3 nights with a glass of milk, then increased to 10 mg and finally 15 mg as the nightly dose. In general, the older the patient, the more responsive she is to sex hormones and stil-boestrol has the advantage over androgens in that they produce no virilisation. Upon failure, 5-FU therapy is employed. With progression, Megace can then be prescribed. With failure, adriamycin may be offered and finally a trial with 5-drug therapy.

It gives much concern to see, as a routine measure, patients with advanced breast cancer treated with a modified Cooper's 5-drug regimen as the initial therapy. There is no question about this producing a higher response than sex hormones or cytotoxic drugs, except perhaps adriamycin. The question that must be asked is what effective therapy can be offered to these patients after failure following several months on this combi-nation. I believe it is doubtful if they would then be responsive to hormonal manipulation, additive or ablative. And, I doubt if they would then respond to any of the drugs singly that are part of the 5-drug combination. I believe it is wrong to employ therapy initially that would compromise responsiveness to other methods upon failure. We are not, with rare exceptions, searching for treatment that produces the highest incidence of response, but rather for a logical sequence of therapy that will yield the longest useful palliation.

The terminal patient

Occasionally a patient with advanced breast cancer when first seen may be in a serious condition such as with bilateral pleural and pericardial malignant effusions, lymphogenous spread to the lung requiring oxygen, or rapidly advancing liver metastases. In such dire situations, 5-drug therapy should be initiated at once in an all-out effort to induce a remission. This will usually occur within 4–5 weeks at which point the 5-drug combination is terminated, and the patient is given a loading course of 5-FU administered by multiple daily doses, then weekly injections. This regimen may well maintain the remission. The reasons for halting the 5-drug therapy if a remission occurs in 4 or 5 weeks is because, with that short exposure to the combination, patients still have a good chance of responding to single drugs given sequentially. It is, furthermore, far less expensive and simpler in terms of toxicity to maintain a patient on 1 drug as compared with the 5-drug combination. If initial treatment with 5-drug therapy given for not more than 5 weeks fails to produce a remission, it should be halted and a trial with adriamycin should be given. If a significant response is induced with this compound, it should then be discontinued due to the ultimate hazard of cardiac toxicity and replaced with 5-FU given as a loading course followed by weekly doses as above.

In summary, in view of the many treatment methods available in disseminated breast cancer, one should never withhold treatment until there is advanced disease. It is far preferable to treat these patients early and in a logical order. Upon failure with one modality, there is nothing to be gained in persisting with that regimen but rather proceed to the next sequence of therapy. In this way, one can hope to improve significantly the lot of the altogether too many women who succumb to advanced breast cancer.

REFERENCES

1. Fisher, B., Slack, N. H., Cavanaugh, P. J., Gardner, B. and Ravdin, R. G. (1970). Postoperative radiotherapy in the treatment of breast cancer: Results of the NSABP clinical trial. *Ann. Surg.*, **172**, 711
2. Fisher, B., Ravdin, R. G., Ausman, R. K., Slack, N. H., Moore, G. E., Noer, R. J. and Cooperating Investigators (1968). Surgical adjuvant chemotherapy in cancer of the breast: Results of a decade of cooperative investigation. *Ann. Surg.*, **168**, 337
3. Ravdin, R. G., Lewison, E. F., Slack, N. H., Dao, T. L., Gardner, B., State, D., Fisher, B. and Cooperating Investigators (1970). Results of a clinical trial concerning the worth of a prophylactic oophorectomy for breast carcinoma. *Surg. Gynecol. Obstet.*, **131**, 1055
4. Fisher, B. (1972). Surgical adjuvant therapy for breast cancer. *Cancer*, **30**, 1556
5. Cooperative Breast Cancer Group (1964). Testosterone propionate therapy in breast cancer. *J. Amer. Med. Ass.*, **188**, 1069
6. Mackman, S., Ramirez, G. and Ansfield, F. J. (1967). Results of 5-fluorouracil (NSC-19893) given by the multiple daily dose method in disseminated breast cancer. *Cancer Chemother. Rep.*, **51**, 483
7. Johnson, E. C., Ansfield, F. J., Ramirez, G. and Davis, H. L., Jr. (1973). Further clinical studies of 5-fluorouracil (5-FU; NSC-19893) given by the multiple daily dose method in disseminated breast cancer. *Cancer Chemother. Rep.*, **57**, 59
8. Ansfield, F. J., Ramirez, G., Mackman, S., Bryan, G. T. and Curreri, A. R. (1969). A ten-year study of 5-fluorouracil in disseminated breast cancer with clinical results and survival times. *Cancer Res.*, **29**, 1062
9. Blomgren, S. E., Wolberg, W. H. and Kisken, W. A. (1965). Effect of fluoropyrimidines on delayed cutaneous hypersensitivity. *Cancer Res.*, **25**, 977
10. Jacobs, E. M., Reeves, W. J., Wood, D. A., Pugh, R., Braunwald, J. and Bateman, J. R. (1971). Treatment of cancer with weekly intravenous 5-FU. *Cancer*, **27**, 1302
11. Personal communication with Dr Emil J. Freireich
12. Cooper, R. G. (1969). Combination chemotherapy in hormone-resistant breast cancer. *Proc. Am. Ass. Cancer Res.*, **10**, 15
13. Ansfield, F. J., Ramirez, G., Korbitz, B. C. and Davis, H. L., Jr. (1971). Five-drug therapy for advanced breast cancer: a phase 1 study. *Cancer Chemother. Rep.*, **55**, 183
14. Goldenberg, I. S., Waters, M. N., Ravdin, R. S., Ansfield, F. J. and Segaloff, A. (1973). Androgenic therapy for advanced breast cancer in women. *J. Amer. med. Ass.*, **223**, 1267

7

Tests of prediction

R. D. Bulbrook

1. Introduction

There are a number of reviews on prognostic factors in breast cancer[1-4] and an excellent book[5]. The fact that some of these references are dated should not deter the reader since progress in the field of prediction is extremely slow and there are very few new well-established findings, although some promising leads are developing. In this Chapter an attempt has been made not only to list the salient findings but to discuss the entire subject of predicting the clinical course of breast cancer as a whole and to point out some of the difficulties that have emerged over the last 20 years. These difficulties ought to have been foreseeable but perhaps this statement stems from hindsight. On the other hand, if workers in the field had realised that they were committing themselves to so difficult a task, it is quite probable that many of them would never have embarked on their research but would have turned their attention to easier fields.

The overall results of the last 20 years' work are depressing. As far as metastatic breast cancer is concerned, there is not a single predictive test that is so firmly established that its use is mandatory. In the strictest scientific sense, there is no definitive proof of the efficacy of the majority of the published methods of prediction and, for this reason, it is perfectly ethical to select particular treatments for patients by the standard clinical methods (precedent or instinct). Even when there is evidence that selection of patients for a particular treatment by means of predictive measurements will lead to a substantial increase in benefit, this is almost certainly accomplished by denying treatment to a small proportion of potential responders. The question of prediction and selection then becomes a subjective one, and every clinician has to make up his own mind about the level of response he requires in his responsive patients and the degree of misclassification he will accept in the light of the severity of the disease and the burden of the proposed treatment.

Prior to 1896, there was no effective treatment for disseminated breast cancer. With the introduction of oöphorectomy by Beatson[6], prediction of response might have been desirable but was clearly not essential since no serious objections have been raised against using this treatment for a hundred patients in order to help thirty. When bilateral adrenalectomy was first used in 1951, and hypophysectomy in 1953, the climate of opinion changed and some surgeons have refused to countenance the use of these treatments on the grounds that the majority of unresponsive patients had to pay too high a price in order that a minority should enjoy a worthwhile remission of their disease. An urgent search for predictive indices started in the early 1950s and is still going on fitfully.

In recent years, there has been a critical reappraisal of the benefits of the treatment of primary breast cancer by radical mastectomy, exemplified by the pessimistic calculations of Zelen[7] whose figures indicated a cure rate of 6%. This questionning has led to clinical trials of less radical surgery[8], counterbalanced by claims for the excellence of even more radical surgery[9].

But in the very long run, it does not seem likely that alterations in surgical techniques for the treatment of the primary disease will have a dramatic effect on mortality (of course, as Lord Keynes pointed out, in the very long run we shall all be dead). No amount of tinkering about with the pectoralis major is going to help a patient, ostensibly in Stage 1 or 2, who has, in reality, systemic disease. The identification of these women is one of the most urgent tasks.

A further reason for developing new methods of prediction of the clinical course of the disease stems from the fact that new methods of treatment are now available. There have already been some attempts to use prophylactic endocrine[10-12] or chemotherapeutic treatments[13] at the time of mastectomy. The present discontent with current therapy for the primary disease will almost inevitably lead to many more of such attempts to alter the clinical course of breast cancer. We can look forward with lively apprehension to a flood of anecdotal accounts of new and bizarre adjuvant therapies and, possibly, a few properly conducted clinical trials.

If adjuvant therapy at the time of mastectomy is to be widely used, efficient predictive tests would be of the greatest possible value. In the advanced, progressive condition, treated by endocrine ablation, responsive patients survive an average of 20 months: unresponsive patients, 10 months[14]. Perhaps 5% will still be in remission five years after operation[15]. In patients with primary disease, however, an obstinate minority survive, disease-free, for 10 years or more, even if they have the gravest prognostic signs at diagnosis[16]. The choice before the clinician is now of an entirely different kind from that facing him in deciding whether to carry out major ablative surgery. It is now whether to treat a number of patients who have been cured by mastectomy with additional endocrine — or chemo-therapy, or possibly, immunotherapy.

2. Basic difficulties in predicting response

It may now be useful to examine why so little has been achieved in predicting the clinical course of breast cancer when it is obvious that there is a necessity for valid predictive tests. The difficulties in devising useful tests have turned out to be formidable: some of them have already been discussed by Bulbrook[17] but it might be helpful to reiterate these and to add some new ones.

The first problem is the heterogeneity of the patients. Most workers accept that this is a grave disadvantage but ignore it. For example, although the majority of patients present with the disease between the ages of 45 to 70 years, it is not uncommon for a normal hospital intake to span a range from 25 to 85 years. Why should the biological factors that determine age at diagnosis and the clinical behaviour of the tumour be constant? Surely, there is evidence that this is not the case. For example, MacMahon and his colleagues[18] have shown in a massive case-control study that early parity is associated with a marked diminution in life-long risk, and it is now common to speak of the "protective effects" of pregnancy. But women who die from breast cancer between the ages of 15 and 24 are more often married and fertile than nulliparous or unmarried[19]. In this small and unusual group of women early pregnancy cannot be protective. Again, hormone responsiveness varies with age: although the effectiveness of androgen therapy may be uniform at all ages[20], the remission rate for oestrogen therapy increases steadily with advancing age after the menopause[21].

The differences in the extent of the disease at first presentation are enormous, ranging from patients with small tumours confined to the breast, with no metastases (evidenced by a survival after mastectomy almost as good as that in the general population[22]) to those with lesions which are inoperable when first seen. Others may have what appears to be very early cancer, but Galasko[23] using gamma camera scintigraphy, has shown that as many as 24% of such patients can be identified as having metastases.

Tumour growth and dissemination rates differ widely: metastases may appear 20 years after mastectomy, whereas Strax & Shapiro[24] found a considerable number of women whose breast cancer developed between annual mammographic and clinical screening, implying a very rapid rate of growth. Doubling times vary between 20 to 200 days and are related to survival after mastectomy[25].

There are 2 logical answers to these problems of excessive variation. The first is to study a relatively homogeneous group of patients, selected on the basis of a carefully designed protocol. The obvious disadvantage here is to find enough such patients in the usual hospital intake. If too few patients are available, the time span for completing the investigation may be so long that changes may occur in the presentation of the disease. Cady[26] reports significant trends towards smaller primary cancers and fewer axillary metastases from 1948 to 1968.

The second answer is to study very large numbers of patients so that the effects of variables such as age, menopausal status, tumour size, nodal involvement, etc. can be analysed. Since few hospitals see enough patients the recent moves to establish international trials involving several thousands of patients is to be welcomed, although these trials in themselves present formidable problems.

The next important problem in establishing effective predictive tests in breast cancer is that of assessing clinical

response. In chorioepithelioma, the excretion of gonadotrophins provide a system for the rapid objective monitoring
of response[27] and this is one of the main reasons why treatment
of this cancer is so successful. There is no such biological marker
in patients with breast cancer. It has taken decades of work to
establish protocols defining objective response to treatment;
these are cumbersome and their use requires a high degree of
clinical skill. Response to most therapies is slow and it may take
a period of 6 weeks before a treatment can be said to have
failed. Six months may be required, with objective signs of
regression and with no new tumours appearing before a treatment can be designated as successful. In spite of widespread
agreement that strict protocols such as those of the American
Cooperative Breast Cancer Group or of Guy's Hospital Breast
Unit[28] are essential, it is still distressingly common to find
authors describing their patients as "well", with no time scale,
or to find reliance placed on such uncertain markers as relief
of pain or diminution of pleural effusions.

Response to treatment is a continuous variable, not an
all-or-none phenomenon and, like survival, is log-normally
distributed. This adds to the difficulties in that most workers
prefer to express their results as "success" or "failure", which
means the introduction of an arbitrary cut-off point varying
from worker to worker. Other problems connected with
measurement of response have been exhaustively discussed by
Brennan[29].

Even with the greatest possible care exercised by experienced workers, the clinical results obtained with small
samples can vary widely. For example, 28 protocol trials were
run using testosterone propionate. Each trial was carried out
on 24 patients. The remission rates varied between 4% and
39%, with an overall mean of 20%[29]. Quite clearly, a predictive test based on various biochemical measurements in a
series of patients with a 39% remission rate might lead to the
conclusion that a highly effective predictor had been found. A
repetition of the test on an apparently identical group of
patients with a 4% rate might well lead to a contrary opinion.

The clinical effectiveness of different hormone treatments
varies widely. All hormonal manoeuvres do not produce a
single standard remission rate and, indeed, may work through

different biological mechanisms. For example, hypophysectomy is more effective than adrenalectomy at Guy's Hospital[30] but there is some evidence that this finding is due to the preferential response to hypophysectomy of women without a previous mastectomy, who do badly when treated by adrenalectomy[31]. It follows that a predictive test that may measure hormone responsiveness (in the broadest and most general sense) may be useful for one treatment and relatively ineffective for another. Yet it is still common to find small series of patients treated with 9 different therapies, with the bland assumption that the agents are identical because they are steroids.

It is also widely and erroneously assumed that when a surgeon says that he has carried out an adrenalectomy or hypophysectomy, all the glandular tissue in question has been removed. Nothing could be further from the truth. Patients who have been treated by oöphorectomy and adrenalectomy, or by hypophysectomy not infrequently continue to excrete appreciable quantities of steroid and polypeptide hormones[32]. Although completeness of operation may not be essential, it would be useful if it were checked by pre- and post-operative hormone assays. Perhaps the availability of simple radioimmunological assays will make this a practicable proposition. Failing this, post-mortem examinations might be salutary. For example, Stretton Young[33] found what appeared to be viable pituitary tissue in all of 14 patients treated with ^{198}Au or ^{90}Y. Obviously, predictive tests are unlikely to function efficiently if there is considerable variation in the amounts of glandular tissue removed at operation.

3. Steps in establishing a valid predictive test

The points discussed above may indicate how difficult it is to establish a realistic predictive test capable of day-to-day use for the generality of patients. There are 3 logical steps that may help to prevent some of the more egregious errors. The first step is the obvious one, where a correlation is sought between whatever predictive variable is chosen and response to a given therapy, in a retrospective investigation. Even this basic step seems to present difficulties. If enough variables are measured, in a small enough series, a perfect separation of responders and non-responders can usually be achieved. But the same degree of separation could probably be achieved by measuring variables such as shoe and hat size. Discriminant function analysis, used unwarily, is a very useful mathematical technique for turning rubbish of this sort into an apparently useful predictive system[34]. The second logical step is, therefore, to use the predictive variables prospectively in some sort of formal trial. There is an ominous lack of papers on this subject, either because investigators cannot be bothered or because their prize predictors simply came apart in their hands. Given the unlikely event of a predictive test surviving this far, the third logical step is to show that a significant increase occurs in the remission rate of patients selected for treatment. There is only 1 paper describing such a method: it is in Japanese[35], lacking a summary in English, and this may explain why so splendid an example has not been widely copied.

An alternative to these steps in checking the usefulness of a predictive system is to hope that other workers will repeat the original work so that a body of experience is accumulated, involving a wide variety of patients and treatments.

4. Stage and grade

The clinical or pathological stage of a patient is so taken for granted that it is usually ignored by workers who are interested in biochemical tests of prediction. Most of them imagine that the only reason for measuring stage is for the benefit of pathologists and statisticians. This was not too unreasonable an opinion in the past since patients with operable breast cancer were all offered identical treatment (radical mastectomy) whatever their stage (1 or 2) or degree of nodal involvement. Yet accurate staging (and to a lesser extent, measurement of tumour grade) provides prognostic information as good as, or better than, that obtained by other methods. What is more, stage and grade may be of critical importance in assessing the usefulness of a predictive test. Consider Cutler's data[36]. The 10-year survival of patients with no nodal involvement is about 70%. If pathological examination reveals metastases in the axillary nodes, survival is about 30%. Now, if the predictive variable is directly related to tumour growth rates and early metastatic spread it would follow that an apparently successful predictive test would result, providing stage is ignored. In other words, it is quite possible that many workers have discovered expensive and complicated biochemical methods of measuring pathological stage.

An abnormality in hormone production or in immune response may be one of the main reasons why a patient presents in a particular stage. That this may be true was hinted at by an early finding of Miller & Durant[37]. They measured urinary androgen and corticosteroid metabolites and showed that the ratio of these 2 groups of steroids fell as stage advanced. Their conclusion was that advancing disease was responsible for endocrine changes. But an alternative explanation is that the abnormal steroid ratio was related to the factors that determine metastatic spread. In a recent study of patients at Guy's Hospital it was found that the lower the excretion of urinary androgens, the more likely it was that a patient would have Stage 2 disease, rather than Stage 1. The results (unpublished observations) are shown in Table 7.1. Obviously, a prospective study of pre-diagnosis androgen excretion would be necessary to resolve this point satisfactorily.

These comments do not apply only to the primary disease but may be apposite in patients with metastatic breast cancer. For example, Myers et al.[38] have shown that the survival of patients with unfavourable status with regard to tumour size, nodal involvement, nuclear grade and sinus histiocytosis is 5 times as bad as that of patients with favourable status. The free interval (the period between mastectomy and recurrence) cannot exceed 2 years for many of the patients with all 4 prognostic signs unfavourable, since about 50% are dead

Table 7.1 RELATION BETWEEN 11-DKS AND PROPORTION OF PRE-MENOPAUSAL PATIENTS WITH BREAST CANCER IN STAGE 1 AND 2 ($n = 182$).

11-DKS (mg/24 h)	Stage 1	Stage 2	% Stage 2
0.0–2.0	20	28	58%
2.1–3.0	22	22	50%
3.1–4.0	22	15	41%
4.1–6.0	20	16	44%
>6.1	10	7	41%

within 3 years. There is almost universal agreement that patients with short free intervals respond badly to endocrine ablation[1-5] and it is, therefore, highly likely that response to ablation is related to the prognostic signs described by Myers et al.[38]. Once again, if the appearance of these grave signs were due to a subnormal androgen production, it would not be surprising if the steroid measurements alone appeared to "predict" response to ablation.

The argument can be taken one stage further. Since the 5-year survival is 76% for patients with negative nodes, compared with 62% for those with 1-3 nodes involved and 35% for those with more than 3 nodes[13] it would not be unreasonable to test predictive methods in patients where the degree of nodal involvement is known.

The same reasoning applies to the grade of malignancy of a tumour, which is also highly related to survival (see, for example, Wolff[39]). The question is how many predictive tests, especially those involving biochemical or histological measurements on the tumour tissue itself (such as oestrogen receptor sites, behaviour in tissue culture, Barr-body counts, etc.) are simply an extremely inefficient and unconscious method for measuring grade?

Incidentally, in the preceding paragraphs, the extent of the disease and its biological characteristics and clinical behaviour have been treated as if they were completely related. This is not necessarily so.

5. Histological predictors

Since we have been dealing with well-established prognostic factors such as stage and grade, it would be as well to describe some newer findings that indicate the potential value of pathological or histological signs.

ELASTOSIS

Breast cancer frequently shows hyalin acellular material in periductal areas or in the carcinoma itself, readily detectable after staining with 2% toluidine blue. Lundmark[40] comments that there is sometimes a very close contact between the carcinoma cells and elastin fibrils, suggesting some kind of relationship between them, possibly that the carcinoma cells may themselves induce the production of elastin.

Shivas & Douglas[41] report a highly significant relation between the degree of elastosis and survival after simple mastectomy and radiotherapy or in patients with recurrence after adrenalectomy. In the former group, patients with no elastosis had a mean survival time of 33 months compared with 94 months for patients with gross elastosis. The mean survival time after mastectomy and later adrenalectomy was 33 months in patients with no elastosis compared with 122 months in those with advanced elastosis.

BARR-BODY COUNTS
Gross and his colleagues[42] reported in 1965 that patients whose tumour cells were of female nuclear sex had a 44% 5-year survival after mastectomy compared with 20% in those with male nuclear sex. In the same year Hienz[43] found that chromatin-positive patients responded better to testosterone or oöphorectomy than a control group whereas these therapies diminished survival in patients who were chromatin-negative. The use of Barr-body counts for prediction of response has been re-examined recently by Perry[44] who found the mean count in 14 responders to hypophysectomy to be about 50 compared with 20 in non-responders. Patients who survived 1–12 months after treatment had a mean count of 18: in those who survived more than 30 months, the mean count was 58. The steroid ratio used by the Hammersmith Hospital for prediction of response to endocrine therapy (which will be discussed in detail subsequently) was measured at the same time. In general, the ratio gave much the same degree of prediction as the Barr-body count but Perry[44] felt that the combination of both variables improved prediction.

NUCLEAR DNA CONTENT
Atkin[45] found two distinct groups, roughly equal in number, in a study of the modal deoxyribonucleic acid values of 67 patients. Patients with near diploid values had a better 8-year survival than those with triploid-tetraploid values. However, this author pointed out a tendency for a relationship between his findings and the degree of histological differentiation of the

tumour, and with nodal involvement, and suggests that both grade and assessment of sex chromatin may give similar predictive results to measurements of DNA.

SINUS HISTIOCYTOSIS

There is still a considerable controversy concerning the usefulness of sinus histiocytosis as a predictive factor which probably stems from the difficulty in interpreting the histological picture. Until this is resolved there is little point in discussing this topic further.

6. Endocrine predictors

Most of the work on prediction of response to treatment has been concentrated on measurements of endocrine function, or of the response of the tumour to hormones (this includes measurement of hormone receptor sites in the tumour and tissue culture techniques). The reason for this is partly historical and partly intuitive. Early work with laboratory animals indicated that large doses of oestrogenic hormones were effective in causing breast cancer in rodents. From such experiments the concept of hormone imbalance as an important factor in the aetiology of the disease developed. The assumption was made, probably subconsciously, that a similar extreme imbalance in the production of endogeneous hormone existed in man and that measurement of hormonal status might therefore provide useful information. A more reasonable concept was that, if the production of a hormone on which tumour growth was thought to depend was subnormal, then it would be extremely unlikely that removal of the gland producing the hormone would lead to regression of the tumour. In other words, hormone tests might identify women with hormone-unresponsive tumours.

OESTROGENS AND PROGESTERONE

The hormones thought to be of greatest importance were the female sex hormones, the oestrogens and progesterone. With the development of reasonable analytical methods from 1955 onwards, these were the target for the first investigations.

Strong and his colleagues[46] were the first to find no significant differences between the amounts of urinary oestrogen metabolites in responders and non-responders to ablative operations. Others had similar findings[47–49].

These and other results were disappointing. There is really no evidence that the amounts of oestrogens excreted in the urine are related in any way to response to endocrine therapy. But the concept that the oestrogens play a key role in the aetiology of human breast cancer and in the control of the rate of tumour growth was so firmly believed that these results were accepted with great reluctance and reasons were sought to set them aside. There was a sterile controversy about the quality of the early oestrogen assays but, valid though some of the criticisms may have been, no correlation was found whatever assay system was used. It was postulated that the urinary metabolites might not reflect plasma levels, in spite of the fact that they correlated with the degree of cornification of the vaginal smear[50]. One point still to be resolved is that the classical urinary oestrogen metabolites (oestrone, oestradiol-17β and oestriol) represent only some 20% of the total oestrogen metabolites in the urine. In endometrial carcinoma, it is claimed that abnormally large amounts of unidentified metabolites appear in the urine[51].

Lemon et al.[52] pointed out that the ratio of urinary oestriol to oestrone and oestradiol is subnormal in women with breast cancer and that normalisation of this ratio by hormonal therapy contributes to the arrest of growth of oestradiol-dependent metastases. They further state that no remissions were found after major surgery unless the ratio rose to a normal value. While there is little evidence that the oestriol ratio is a reliable guide to clinical course, there is at least the possibility that it may be related to the differences between the incidence rates in Japan and America[53]. If true, this finding is not only of importance in terms of aetiological factors but may have relevance to the clinical course of the disease in that breast cancer in Japan runs a more benign course than the disease in Western countries[54].

An ingenious test was suggested by Shucksmith, Bonser, Dossett, Henderson & Jull[55]. They assessed biopsy material from the unaffected breast and graded it as stimulated or unstimulated. At the same time urinary oestrogen excretion was measured. Four combinations of the parameters were possible. With low oestrogen excretion (less than 3 μg/24 h of oestrone, plus oestradiol, plus oestriol) and unstimulated breast tissue, no response to either hypophysectomy or adrenalectomy was predicted. The second category was a low oestrogen excretion in conjunction with stimulated breast tissue: here, a response to hypophysectomy was expected. The third category was a high oestrogen excretion with unstimulated breast tissue: a response to adrenalectomy was predicted. With a high oestrogen excretion and stimulated breast tissue, either operation was expected to succeed. In a series of 18 patients, this test led to a correct prediction of response in 14 instances. The results are shown in Table 7.2.

Table 7.2 PREDICTION OF RESPONSE TO ENDOCRINE ABLATION USING OESTROGEN EXCRETION AND HISTOLOGICAL EXAMINATION OF TISSUE FROM BREAST BIOPSY (SHUCKSMITH *ET AL.*[55]).

	Response	Expected	Observed
Adrenalectomy	Remission	10	7
	Failure	5	4
Hypophysectomy	Remission	2	2
	Failure	1	1

This was a remarkable piece of work for its time. It was not then widely appreciated that prolactin was a hormonal carcinogen in mice[56] and that the DMBA-induced tumour in the rat was prolactin-dependent rather than oestrogen-dependent[57]. Incidentally, the finding of a low oestrogen excretion in conjunction with a stimulated breast tissue in some cases provides a physiological explanation for the failure of urinary oestrogen assays alone to provide predictive information. The clear inference is that hormones other than oestrogens are responsible for the stimulation. On balance, the weight of the evidence is that oestrogen assays alone provide little or no prognostic information. If there is a real relationship between oestrogen stimulation and tumour growth, it must be so subtle that the usual methods of measuring oestrogen status will not detect it.

Very little work has been done on plasma progesterone levels or on the possible prognostic use of measurements of the main urinary metabolite pregnanediol and the results are inconclusive.

PROLACTIN AND GROWTH HORMONE

While the majority of workers undertook investigations into the role of oestrogens in the aetiology and clinical course of breast cancer in the late 1950s, a few pioneers turned their attention to the protein hormones of the anterior pituitary. Growth hormone and prolactin had long been known to be mammogenic in many animal species[58] but assays suitable for measuring growth hormone in man were not available and the existence of a distinct human prolactin was in doubt. Early work depended on bio-assays and the inevitable controversy developed. Hadfield[59] found a correlation between the results of his assay (which depended on breast growth in hypophysectomised weanling male mice primed with oestrogen and progesterone) and response to hypophysectomy. Others did not[60,61].

McCalister and Welbourne[62] in 1962, administered ovine prolactin to 10 patients with metastatic breast cancer and measured calcium excretion. In 4 patients who failed to respond to hypophysectomy, calcium excretion did not change but in 6 patients who responded, calcium excretion increased markedly.

At this stage the interest in prolactin quietly died, but in 1970 Boot[56] published a splendid review indicating that prolactin was a potent carcinogen in mice. Pearson and his colleagues[57] showed that the DMBA-induced rat tumour was dependent not on oestrogen but on prolactin and suggested that the rat system was "a model for man". Shortly afterwards, evidence for the existence of a separate human prolactin molecule was obtained and the way was open for the establishment of a specific radioimmunoassay[63].

Boyns and his colleagues[64] measured plasma levels of prolactin against a standard made from amniotic fluid. The mean plasma levels and standard deviations in controls and patients with benign breast disease, primary breast cancer, advanced local disease and advanced general disease were identical. At first sight this is a somewhat disappointing finding since it would mean that if prolactin levels were to be of predictive value, one might expect to be dealing with values lying within a fairly narrow normal range. However, their normal range (which was expressed in logarithms) was enormous. In the controls the 95% limits lay between 3 and 200 milliampoules/ml. With a 70-fold difference between values in individual patients it would be interesting to know whether those at either end of the range responded differently to endocrine therapy. One might expect that patients producing little or no prolactin would not respond to hypophysectomy but objective remissions can occur in patients with extremely high plasma prolactin levels following stalk section[65].

Growth hormone is also mammotrophic in some species but it seems unlikely to be important in this respect in man. The availability of a good radioimmunological assay led to some investigations in patients with breast cancer with results that are difficult to interpret. Pearson et al.[66] found a paradoxical hypersecretion of growth hormone in response to a glucose load in 9 of his 23 patients. Greenwood et al.[67] reported a similar finding. Both groups stated that the well-documented abnormalities in carbohydrate metabolism in patients with breast cancer could not be explained on the basis of their growth hormone assay results. There is no information concerning the prognostic significance of these findings but it seems unlikely that the assays would be informative with so variable a response.

CORTICOSTEROIDS

Early investigations of adrenal cortex function in breast cancer relied on the somewhat insensitive method of measurement of urinary 17-hydroxycorticosteroid (17-OHCS). With one exception[68], raised levels were found in patients with metastatic disease[69,70]. Jensen and her colleagues[71] extended these studies by measuring production and clearance rates of cortisol. The latter were normal in both 8 early and 9 advanced cases but the production rate was significantly raised in the advanced cases. The raised production rate appears to be a result of a defect in adrenal steroidogenesis in which more substrate is converted into cortisol and less into androgens than in normal women[72,73].

The high cortisol production appears to be related to a poor prognosis but the connection is tenuous[74].

Perhaps the most thorough study of cortisol production in relation to the clinical course of the disease is that by Saez[75]. Cortisol production rates were measured in 31 patients with breast cancer, under basal conditions and with dexamethasone suppression. The production rate was normal for patients with primary disease and no evidence of recurrence. In patients with advanced disease, the rate increased and suppression of cortisol secretion with dexamethasone was less effective. There was evidence that patients with a poor response to treatment (which was not detailed) showed the least depression with dexamethasone. Bishop & Ross[76] made a similar finding in that failure of suppression measured by plasma 11-hydroxy-corticosteroid changes was associated with poor prognosis in lung cancer.

Ghosh, Lockwood and Pennington[77] have recently found that the urinary excretion of corticosteroid sulphates was raised in patients with breast cancer: if metastases were present a more marked increase in excretion was found. These authors quote the work of Dao[78], on the ability of tumour cells to sulphate steroids, and suggest that the amount of corticosteroid sulphate in the urine may be related to metastatic spread of the disease.

ANDROGENS

The first chemical method for the assay of urinary androgen metabolites measured the 17-oxosteroids (17-KS) as a group. Many of these compounds were not derived from androgenic precursors but from corticosteroids and the interpretation of the results was difficult. Nevertheless, early studies indicated that 17-KS excretion was subnormal in patients with breast cancer. Unfortunately, similar results were found in a wide variety of serious chronic illnesses[79] and the findings in breast cancer were ascribed to non-specific effects of debilitating diseases.

In 1957, Allen et al.[80] carried out a partial fractionation of the 17-KS and showed that patients who excreted more 11-deoxy-17-oxosteroids (derived from androgenic precursors) relative to the amounts of 11-oxy-17-oxosteroids had a better response to adrenalectomy or hypophysectomy than patients in whom the ratio was reversed. Subsequently, further fractionation of the 11-deoxy-17-oxosteroid fraction showed that patients responsive to endocrine ablation tended to excrete larger amounts of dehydroepiandrosterone, androsterone and aetiocholanolone than unresponsive patients. Furthermore, the latter patients excreted larger amounts of 17-OHCS, and a ratio of aetiocholanolone to 17-OHCS appeared to separate the two clinical groups successfully. A discriminant function was calculated which appeared to divide responsive and unresponsive patients effectively. The discriminant was

80 − 80 (17-OHCS, mg/24 h) + aetiocholanolone (μg/24 h)

When the assay results were substituted in the formula, patients excreting large amounts of aetiocholanolone relative to the 17-OHCS had "positive discriminants" and conversely, patients excreting small amounts of aetiocholanolone relative to the 17-OHCS had "negative discriminants". The remission rate for adrenalectomy or hypophysectomy was significantly higher in patients with positive discriminants than in those with negative discriminants[81]. The main weight of the predictive power of the discriminant was carried by the androgen factor.

These investigations contained most of the faults outlined in the beginning of this chapter and the main problem was how much reliance could be placed on the findings. It had been shown that hypophysectomy was significantly more effective than adrenalectomy, at Guy's Hospital, but there were insufficient facilities to offer all patients the better treatment. A prospective trial was started in which all patients with positive discriminants were offered hypophysectomy, in the expectation of a high remission rate. Patients with negative discriminants were offered adrenalectomy since it was felt that they could not be abandoned on the basis of an unproven biochemical test. The results of this first prospective trial were that the remission rate for hypophysectomy doubled (46% against 23%) while that for patients treated by adrenalectomy was only 9%[82]. This was unacceptable, and the trial was stopped. Even at this stage, there was still a justifiable reluctance to rely on the discriminant. A second prospective study was therefore undertaken in which patients with negative discriminants were treated by hypophysectomy and those with positive discriminants, by adrenalectomy. The response to adrenalectomy tripled to 30% but response to hypophysectomy in patients with negative discriminants was at the borderline of acceptability, at 13%[83].

It was at this stage that it became obvious that variables other than androgen and corticoid metabolite excretion were important in relation to response and that these variables affected the predictive power of the discriminant. Chief among them were menopausal status and free period. Women up to 6 years after the menopause, with negative discriminants, had a very low response rate (some 5%) and those with a free interval of less than 2 years suffered in the same way. There was evidence that mastectomy status was important in that patients who had been previously treated by mastectomy fared better at adrenalectomy than those who had not[31].

To summarise; a significant relationship had been demonstrated between response to endocrine ablation and the urinary excretion of androgen and corticosteroid metabolites. What was not determined was the precise relationship between the discriminant and other predictive variables.

Armitage et al.[84] looked into this problem using a computer programme in which a series of dichotomies were made, using the most effective predictors first and the least effective last. Starting with 28 variables, a large number of categories of patients was formed with very few dichotomies. The response rates of some groups were very high (for example all 7 women in the group "Hypophysectomy — positive discriminant — osseous metastases" responded to treatment) but the numbers of patients in any one group were too small for any degree of certainty. Another approach used by these authors has been to work out the probability of remission for each patient on the basis of hormone-assay results. This seems a most promising method since it offers the clinician more latitude in deciding whether to use endocrine ablation in any particular case. Sarfaty & Tallis[85] developed this idea further and showed that a considerable improvement in prediction could be made by computing the probability of a successful response for a given numerical value of the discriminant. They also showed that a substitution of free period for the 17-OHCS value might improve predictive accuracy in women aged more than 60 years.

Wilson and his colleagues[86] have also used a discriminant function based on ACTH-stimulated levels of urinary 17-OHCS and 17-KS and the free period. The masin predictive variable was the 17-KS component. They found a correct prediction in 18 of 23 responders and 22 of 26 failures[87].

Wilson et al.[88] have described an increase in remission rate if 5-fluorouracil is given immediately after adrenalectomy. All patients who were expected to respond on the basis of their discriminant function did so but half of the patients expected to fail responded to the new combined treatment.

Other workers have also found the urinary androgen excretion, either alone or in combination with 17-OHCS values, to be of predictive significance. Juret et al.[89] had a response rate to ^{90}Y implantation in the pituitary of some 60% in patients who excreted large amounts of androsterone and aetiocholanolone. Kumaoka et al.[90] showed a remarkable correlation between response to adrenalectomy and androgen excretion in Japanese patients. These workers have also demonstrated a substantial and sustained increase in remission rate now that they used the androgen assays for the selection of patients for treatment[35]. At the Hammersmith Hospital[91], a ratio of 17-oxogenic steroids to 11-deoxy-17-oxosteroids is used. In patients with a ratio of more than 9, the response rate was 13% compared with 38% in patients with a ratio of less than 9.

Finally, Sarfaty, Tallis & Pitt[92] have recently reported that total 11-deoxy-17-oxosteroid and aetiocholanolone glucosiduronate levels are significantly lower in women not responding to adrenalectomy compared with those in responders. The sulphates of these steroids and also of androsterone, were also significantly subnormal. Their paper also provides an illuminating discussion of the problems of assessing response and of the usefulness of discriminant function analysis.

It is a pity that such uncharacteristic unanimity is marred by two investigations in which no correlation was found between response and androgen excretion[93-95].

Attempts have been made to use the discriminant function of Bulbrook et al.[81] for prognosis in the early disease. It was claimed originally that patients who had negative discriminants 10 days after mastectomy had a more rapid recurrence rate than those with positive discriminants[96] and that prediction by the discriminant was independent of stage and grade. The 5-year survival in 37 patients with positive discriminants treated by mastectomy was 75%, compared with 50% in 34 cases with negative discriminants[97]. This paper is noteworthy for a splendid misprint; the life-table starts with all patients dead and shows a steady resurrection rate with time.

There now exists a state of considerable confusion and acrimony about steroid excretion in the early disease and the possible prognostic significance. Miller & Durant[37] found fewer women with negative discriminants at diagnosis than did Bulbrook et al.[96]. The latter workers have now accumulated many more patients and agree with Miller & Durant[37] that the proportion of women with negative discriminants is smaller than originally thought[98]. Wade and his colleagues[99] came to the conclusion that the variation in the values for the discriminant in controls (sick and well) and in patients with early breast cancer was so large that it seemed unlikely to be a specific feature of such patients.

Similar findings were made by Cameron and his colleagues[100] who also found no difference between androgen excretion in patients with early breast cancer and controls. The controversy concerning the normality of steroid excretion in patients at diagnosis remains to be resolved but, whatever the outcome, it does not necessarily affect the possible prognostic value of such measurements. In a recent report[98] 50% of pre-menopausal patients in Stage 2, with negative discriminants had a recurrence in 12 months compared with 40 months for those with positive discriminants; those excreting amounts of aetiocholanolone below 800 μg/24 h (as do some normal women) had twice the recurrence rate of those excreting more than this amount. Other data[98] indicate a similar relationship between plasma dehydroepiandrosterone sulphate levels and recurrence. What is now required is a re-evaluation of the possible relationship between steroid excretion and recurrence rates. For this to be useful, the patients would need to be analysed by menopausal status, stage and grade. This means the accumulation of a large series and even then, a considerable follow-up since the recurrence rate in Stage 1 patients is low. Yet women with Stage 1 disease which is likely to recur are precisely the type of patient we need to identify with accuracy if adjuvant therapy is to be used.

Receptor sites

Hormone responsive tissues such as the uterus, vagina and breast contain specific proteins which have a striking affinity for oestrogens. These components have been called "oestrogen receptors" and it now appears that the first step in oestrogen action involves binding to a receptor[101].

The first indication that the specific uptake of oestrogen by tumour tissue might be related to response to treatment came from a brief report by Folca, Glascock & Irvine[102] who administered tritium-labelled hexoestrol to 10 patients before adrenalectomy. The ratio of counts in tumour compared with those in muscle was determined and in 4 patients, a high ratio (>3.0) was associated with response to adrenalectomy and 6 patients with a ratio of less than 3.0 failed to respond.

Specific oestrogen binding-site measurements in rat and mouse tumours showed that the presence of receptor sites was associated with hormone dependency[103,104].

There has been a number of similar studies in women with breast cancer. James et al.[105] measured oestradiol uptake in 31 patients (aged 29 to 91 years!) and also urinary 17-OHCS and androgens. They found no correlation between the two indices of responsiveness. Since the frequency of positive oestrogen binding increases with age[106] while androgen excretion falls[107] the calculation of a correlation coefficient of oestrogen uptake on steroid excretion seems fraught with uncertainty.

Braunsberg and her colleagues[108] used a 3 hour constant infusion of tritiated oestradiol and measured the ratio of the radioactivity in the tumour to that in the plasma as a measure of tumour uptake. They studied 172 patients with breast cancer, 35 of whom had a recurrence of their disease and were treated by endocrine means. They found what they termed "no unequivocal relation" between oestradiol uptake and response to oöphorectomy, oestrogen or androgen therapy. Objective remissions were found in patients with low or high oestradiol uptake. Although these authors found that a low oestradiol uptake was invariably associated with failure to respond to endocrine ablation, there were only 4 such cases in a series of 18. Two similar patients with an extremely low uptake responded well to oestrogen administration.

Other papers may be found in the literature, in which the workers fail to conform with any of the established protocols for defining response. The uncertain value of such work makes it unnecessary to discuss them here.

In marked contrast to some of the anecdotal results in the literature, Engelsman and his colleagues[109] have convincing evidence of an association between the effects of endocrine therapy and the presence or absence of receptor site. Their patients were 9 pre-menopausal women treated by oöphorectomy and 28 post-menopausal women given the oestrogen antagonist, Nafoxidine (U11100). The clinical response was properly evaluated using the European Co-operative Breast Cancer Group protocol. Of the 17 patients with demonstrable receptor sites in their tumours, 14 had an objective remission of their disease (i.e. some 80%). Of the 20 receptor negative cases, only 2 responded. In a small series, a measured 10% response rate may be far from the true response rate and in the long run it may be that the true rate is much greater than 10%. Jensen and his colleagues have published reports on the association between oestrogen receptors and hormone dependency from time to time over the last few years. Their latest summary deals with 108 women with primary tumours and 51 patients with metastatic breast cancer. About half of the patients' primary tumours contained receptor protein. The advanced patients were treated with 7 different therapies. Eleven of 14 patients with positive receptor sites responded to treatment compared with only 1 of 32 with negative sites[110].

In an earlier report[111], a surprising number of "surgical casualties" were found among women with positive receptor sites (5 out of 14, 36%!) compared with only one casualty in 19 in women with negative sites. It goes without saying that if casualties were called failures, the efficiency of prediction by receptor site assays would be less striking.

The findings of Wittliff et al.[112] show that receptor sites are found more often in post-menopausal than in pre-menopausal women (60% and 30% respectively). These authors discuss extensively and optimistically the possible use of receptor site assays for the prediction of response to endocrine ablation. Yet there is no convincing evidence that more post-menopausal women respond to adrenalectomy or hypophysectomy than pre-menopausal women. Nor is there any reliable evidence that remission rates of 60% can be obtained in any series of patients and it therefore follows that this test will probably give a very considerable number of false positives in post-menopausal patients.

This brief review of receptor site measurements and prognosis shows that there are several inconsistencies in the data. Once again, more evidence is required before one joins in the general euphoria about the usefulness of such measurements, and such evidence would be best obtained by a properly designed multicentre trial rather than by the slow assemblage of individual efforts.

Response of hormones of breast cancer tissue in culture

Mioduszewska et al.[113] studied the effects of various hormones added to both cell and organ cultures of human breast tissue. The hormones used were prolactin, growth hormone, oestradiol-17β, progesterone, testosterone and cortisol. The response to hormones was graded as survival, proliferation, secretion or necrosis. All the hormones used appeared to stimulate some of the cultures. Most effective were prolactin and cortisol. Lack of response to prolactin coupled with stimulation by cortisol was stated to be related to a poor prognosis (after mastectomy or ^{90}Y-implantation). A positive response to prolactin, irrespective of the cortisol was associated with a good prognosis.

Salih, Flax & Hobbs[114] cultured tissue from 14 breast cancers in Trowell's T_8 medium, with different concentrations of oestradiol. They claim that "at least 2 distinct classes of breast tumours" could be identified on the basis of histological appearances and dehydrogenase activity. One class required oestrogen for survival and the other did not, and oestrogen dependence in culture correlated with the clinical response to therapy. In 7 "oestrogen-dependent" cases, 5 different treatments were given; 2 patients were untreated. In the 7 "independent" cases 6 different treatments were applied: one patient was untreated. In 5 instances the clinical response was designated as "well". Some patients had extensive metastases; some had none. No time scales were included so that statements such as "excellent remission until nodes recurred" have no real meaning. It should not be necessary to tabulate the criticisms of such an approach. Stoll[115] has pointed at some of the objections to this work.

A further paper by Flax et al.[116] has raised another anguished and valid criticism from Heuson & Tagnon[117].

Tryptophan metabolism

The amino acid, tryptophan, is an important precursor of nicotinic acid and 5-hydroxytryptamine. Some 16 important metabolites of tryptophan have been isolated from urine and the amounts excreted have been shown to be abnormal in a wide variety of diseases. Of more immediate importance, certain steps in the metabolic pathways are affected profoundly by hormones. For example, tryptophan oxygenase activity is affected by oestrogens, androgens, and corticosteroids.

Rose[118,119] reported that about half of his patients studied after mastectomy excreted elevated amounts of one or more metabolites (3-hydroxy-kynurenine, L-kynurenine, 3-hydroxyanthranilic acid and xanthurenic acid) after a 5 g loading dose of tryptophan. Ten of 18 women with untreated breast cancer showed the same abnormality and Rose suggested that this was due to an increased oestrogenic stimulus arising from an enhanced oestrogenic production or an impaired secretion of androgens. Davis et al.[120] subsequently showed that abnormal tryptophan-metabolite excretion was associated with a reduction in the excretion of urinary aetiocholanolone, and Bell et al.[121] had similar findings. It followed that measurement of tryptophan metabolism might be of prognostic significance. Bell and her colleagues[122] have reported that pre-menopausal patients who excreted small amounts of metabolites had a more rapid recurrence rate than those excreting large amounts (i.e., above the median excretion value for the total group of patients). The rate in the former patients was 35% in 2 years compared with 5% in the latter. No such relationship was found in the post-menopausal women.

Davis & Brown[123] found that patients with abnormal

tryotophan metabolism did not respond to oöphorectomy or oestrogen treatment.

In further studies, Davis et al.[124] examined tryptophan metabolism in 5 patients with early disease, 20 patients with advanced disease, and 25 controls. All were given a 2 g loading dose. Twelve of the 25 patients showed significantly elevated levels of 2 or more metabolites. Most of the abnormalities were found in patients with visceral metastases but it may be important that 2 of the 5 patients with no evidence of metastases also showed an abnormal excretion. The excretion of aetiocholanolone was significantly subnormal in patients with visceral disease.

The position has been made more complicated by a recent finding of Rose & Randall[125]. They showed that patients with bone metastases did not show the expected increase in tryptophan metabolite excretion: the values were identical to those in normal controls. Abnormally high values were found in the majority of patients with soft tissue metastases. This finding correlates well with the observations of Cameron and his colleagues[100] that androgen excretion was normal in women with bone secondaries but depressed in women with local recurrence. Bell (personal communication) has recently studied the predictive value of the levels of the 4 metabolites listed above, in pre- and post-menopausal women, with Stage 1 or 2 tumours, treated by mastectomy. In pre-menopausal women, irrespective of stage, there is a significant relationship between recurrence rate and the amount of 3-HK or L-K excreted. High values run with a good prognosis. In post-menopausal women, high values of 3-HA are associated with a slow recurrence rate.

Enzymes

Hilf[126] has studied enzyme activities in a variety of animal tumours and in human infiltrating ductal carcinoma. Some 27% of the latter had a ratio of glucose-6-phosphate dehydrogenase to α-glycerolphosphate dehydrogenase activities comparable with that in the HMC, 13762M and 13762F transplantable tumours in the rat. The first 2 of these tumours are hormone-independent; the 13762F is not hormone-dependent but hormone-responsive. A further 33% of the human tumours had ratios comparable with those in the R3230AC, MCA and E-line tumours (the first 2 are hormone-responsive; the E-line is oestradiol-dependent). The remaining 40% of human tumours were comparable with the DMBA rat tumour and the T-P line: the former is a mixture of hormone-dependent and responsive growths: the latter is androgen-dependent. Hilf's results[126] indicate that there are at least 3 enzymic patterns in human tumours, each associated with animal models in which the tumours exhibit widely different biological properties. The implication of these results is that there may be multiple pathways to carcinogenesis, leading to multiple tumour types.

Smith et al.[127] measured lactic dehydrogenase, 6-phosphogluconate dehydrogenase and phosphohexose isomerase activities in primary tumours. Patients with free periods in excess of 3 years had lower enzyme activities than those with recurrence within this time. They have evidence for a bimodal distribution of the phosphohexose isomerase/acidic nuclear protein ratio and suggest that patients with low ratios may have hormone responsive tumours.

Dao & Libby[128,129] have studied the ability of tumour tissue to sulphate steroids, especially oestradiol (E2) and dehydroepiandrosterone (DHEA). Of 79 patients treated by adrenalectomy, 27 had tumours that sulphated neither steroid and no responses were obtained. In 27 patients whose tumours sulphated DHEA more efficiently than E2, response to abla-tion was rare (11%) whereas when the ratio of activities was reversed (DHEA/E2 > 1) 81% of the patients responded (17 out of 23).

They also found that their ratio appeared to correlate with recurrence rates after mastectomy, a low ratio being associated with rapid recurrence.

Immunological tests

The concept that cancer may develop from a breakdown in immunological surveillance has led to intensive investiga-tions[130,131]. In general, the evidence is strongest for such an association in cancer of the lymphatic system but some work has been done on patients with breast cancer (admirably summarised by Mackay & Baum[132]).

There is some degree of unanimity that the delayed hypersensitivity response is diminished in patients with breast cancer. Hughes & Mackay[133] found a decrease in response to tuberculin which became more marked as the disease became disseminated. Similar findings were made with intradermal streptokinase-streptodonase (Varidase) solution as the antigen[134]. Poor immune response was associated with short survival[132].

Mitchell[135] also used Varidase and found that the proportion of negative responders was some 3 times greater in patients compared with controls. He found no correlation between the results of Varidase test and the degree of sinus histiocytosis, lymphocytic involvement, or Scarff grading and concluded that the test was not a reliable guide to the accepted histological criteria of host-defence reactions.

Jacobs, Houri, Landon & Merrett[136] determined the circulating levels of immunoglobulin E (IgE) by radioimmunoassay and by radial immunodiffusion. They found low or undetectable levels of this immunoglobulin in most of a group of untreated patients with advanced cancer (which included cases of breast cancer). In the remainder, very high values were recorded which were explained by the presence of an inhibitor. This was sometimes present in the venous drainage of some tumours before it could be detected in peripheral blood. In spite of scathing criticism by Augustin & Chandvadasa[137] (who also found low IgE levels in age-matched noncancer patients in a surgical ward), the simplicity and ease of the assay of Jacobs et al.[136] would make it a relatively simple matter to investigate its usefulness in prediction. The high "inhibitor" levels are not found in treated cancer and it is at least possible that the presence of inhibitor might precede clinical signs of renewed tumour growth.

The use of measurements of foetal antigens in the diagnosis and clinical management of cancer has been reviewed by Laurence & Munro Neville[138]. Almost all tumours possess new antigens which appear to be absent from normal tissues. In addition, many tumours show "retrogenic expression", a term that describes the re-appearance of embryo-specific materials (Stonchill & Bendick[139]).

Laurence & Munro Neville[138] summarised the current literature on carcinoembryonic antigen (CEA) in patients with breast cancer. Of 159 patients examined, 82 (52%) had positive plasma values compared with 0.3% in controls, 4% in benign breast tumours and 7% in fibroadenosis. The percentage of positive tests increased markedly in metastatic disease from 32% in primary breast cancer to 65% in the advanced disease. Lo Gerfo[140] measured carcinoembryonic antigen (CEA) by radioimmunoassay and found 5 of 20 patients in Columbia Stage A had elevated levels, 3 of 10 in Stage B, 1 of 3 in Stage C, and 25 of 30 in Stage D. He suggested that his assay might distinguish between those patients in an early clinical stage but with pathologically advanced disease from patients who had a truly early disease. MacSween et al.[141] used whole serum in their radioimmunoassay and found 11 of 14 patients with breast cancer had levels in excess of 5 ng/ml (that is, above normal levels).

Laurence & Munro Neville[138] are pessimistic about the use of assays of CEA in screening but suggest that the assays may be valuable in monitoring therapy, in that residual disease or the development of metastases might be detectable.

An antigen prepared from a cell line obtained from a pleural effusion of a breast cancer patient was found to be highly reactive against 24 sera obtained from 92 patients with the disease and it was suggested that the complement-fixation test might be useful for screening purposes[142].

Whittaker & Clark[143] showed that the transformation of lymphocytes from peripheral blood into large blast cells was diminished in patients with breast cancer. In normal women some 40% of cells are transformed: in Stages 1 and 2 this drops to about 25% and is slightly lower in Stages 3 and 4. There was almost a complete separation between transformation rates in patients with recurrent disease; patients who were apparently free from disease 1 year or more after treatment had a normal transformation rate whereas those who had failed to respond had a marked depression of transformation.

It is apparent that immunological techniques hold out great promise for future use in prognosis. It would be of the greatest possible value to have a means for the specific detection

of residual tumour cells for the reasons set out at length in the
introduction to this chapter.

End-organ response: sebum production

Measurement of tryptophan metabolism is based on the
premise that the net action of a complicated hormonal milieu
on a target organ can be assessed without the necessity of
multiple endocrine measurements. Another "end-organ"
assay involves the production of sebum which is high in patients
with breast cancer[144,145]. This finding might imply a high
androgen production in spite of all the evidence against this
from direct measurement of urinary and plasma androgens.
Wang et al.[146] found, however, that the high production was
not associated with raised levels of plasma 17-oxosteroids and
attempted to explain this paradoxical finding by postulating
either that there was an increase in end-organ sensitivity in the
patients or that a pituitary factor is involved. As a general
principle, it might be valuable to extend such studies in patients
with breast cancer, looking for possible discrepancies between
direct hormone measurements and end-organ responses. That
described above might prove valuable in increasing the pre-
cision of tests of prediction based on androgen measurements
since it is quite possible that patients who appear to be identical
with regard to androgen status might vary widely in terms of
biological response.

Blood groups

There is considerable literature concerning the preponderance
of blood group A in patients with cancer. Lee[147] summarises
the literature and reports that of 87 patients treated by
oöphorectomy with or without adrenalectomy or with androgens, patients with blood group O had an 11% remission rate
compared with 23% in group A and 36% in group B and
37% in group AB. One cannot help warming to an author who
concludes his article by saying "It is with trepidation that the
data in this article are presented for publication". Anderson[148]
has identified at least 2 types of breast cancer in genetic studies.
One is characterised by early onset, a preponderance of blood
group O, and a high frequency of bilateral disease. The second
occurs more frequently in association with blood group A, is

unilateral, and occurs later in life. There may be a third sporadic type in women with no family history of the disease.

That the controversy over blood groups and cancer is not over is shown by the current disagreement concerning the MNS system (Morosini *et al.*[149]). Irrespective of an abnormal distribution in cancer patients, it would be interesting to check whether this system has prognostic value in view of Lee's work[147].

Factors operating before diagnosis of breast cancer

Haenszel[150] posed the question "Do the forces which influence the rate of tumour induction persist past that point to affect the subsequent course of the disease in the host?" It would be easy to answer this question if we knew anything about the inducing forces. Nevertheless, there are indications that some factors in the pre-cancer period do influence survival when the disease is discovered. One of these is previous pelvic surgery. Not only does oöphorectomy reduce incidence but it also appears to increase survival if breast cancer does develop (MacKay & Sellar[151]; MacMahon *et al.*[152]). Other studies have shown no correlation between survival and socio-economic status and age at birth of first child (Morrison *et al.*[153]).

The second factor is benign breast disease. The controversy concerning the possibility of an increased risk of breast cancer by women with various forms of benign breast disease has been brilliantly reviewed[154]. Silverburg, Chitale & Levitt[155] claim that there is some evidence that mammary cancer associated with concurrent or previous benign breast disease (predominantly fibrocystic disease) may have a better prognosis compared with that of patients whose malignancy is not associated with the benign condition. In their own series of 398 mastectomies they found marginally better nodal status and survival in breast cancer patients with concomitant fibrocystic disease. Brennan *et al.*[156] found that some young women with benign breast disease excreted subnormal amounts of androgen metabolites and had subnormal plasma levels of dehydroepiandrosterone sulphate. Unless the production of androgen subsequently increased, it might be expected that such patients would have a particularly bad prognosis in view of the data associating subnormal androgen production with rapid recurrence after mastectomy, and with hormone-unresponsive tumours.

Izuo et al.[157] measured the nuclear DNA content in hyperplastic lesions from 15 cases of cystic disease of the breast, 8 of whom subsequently developed breast cancer. In these women, an aneuploid DNA distribution was found in 3 whereas the distribution was diploid-to-tetraploid in the 7 women who did not develop breast cancer. They suggest that nuclear DNA measurements might be useful for prognosis in benign disease. The aneuploidy might indicate an unfavourable clinical course in these patients.

Finally, Bulbrook, Hayward & Spicer[158] found that a subnormal excretion of androgens in ostensibly normal women was associated with an enhanced risk of breast cancer. Again, this abnormality may well be associated with a bad prognosis if breast cancer developed.

While there is little information at the moment concerning factors operating before the disease is manifest, the situation may change in the next decade since several prospective studies are in progress which might reveal useful predictive information.

Conclusions

There are, almost certainly, multiple factors involved in the aetiology and clinical course of breast cancer and no single factor is so important that it overrides all others. This review has dealt mainly with endocrine status but viral infection and immune response may be equally important. If there are multiple factors involved, then we may need multiple tests of prediction.

It would not be too difficult to run a simultaneous battery of endocrinological, biochemical, immunological and viral tests on a sufficient number of patients. Given very accurate identification of women at high risk of recurrence in Stage 1 and 2, it might be possible to push ahead vigorously with new forms of adjuvant therapy instead of feeling the way forward cautiously. In the advanced disease, it would be a great relief to use major endocrine surgery only for those with a 90% or 95% chance of a substantial remission of their disease. While it might be a rather disconcerting thought that there would be little to offer patients rejected by accurate testing, at least such tests would clear the way for new efforts in palliation, such as multiple drug chemotherapy.

In the long run, effective treatment for breast cancer will no doubt evolve without any predictive tests at all. But the time taken to reach this state would be dramatically shortened if effective tests could be developed.

ACKNOWLEDGEMENTS

I am very much indebted to the Editor and Mr J. L. Hayward, FRCS, for their advice, and to Mrs R. Walter for her help in preparing this chapter.

REFERENCES

1. Bulbrook, R. D. and Strong, J. A. (1959). *Hormone Studies in Breast Cancer*, p. 215. *Cancer*, Vol. **6**. (R. W. Raven, editor.) London: Butterworth

2. Hall, T. C. (Editor) (1971). Prediction of Response in Cancer Therapy. *Nat. Cancer Inst. Monogr.*, **34**

3. Bulbrook, R. D. (1965). Hormone assays in human breast cancer. *Vitamins & Hormones*, **23**, 329

4. Fairgrieve, J. (1965). Selective criteria for surgical removal of the endocrine glands in advanced breast cancer. *Surgery Gynec. Obstet.*, **120**, 371

5. Forrest, A. P. M. and Kunkler, P. B. (1968). (Editors), *Prognostic Factors in Breast Cancer*. Edinburgh and London: E. & S. Livingstone Ltd

6. Beatson, G. T. (1896). On the treatment of inoperable cases of carcinoma of the mamma: suggestions for a new method of treatment with illustrative cases. *Lancet*, **ii**, 104

7. Zelen, M. (1968). A hypothesis for the natural time history of breast cancer. *Cancer Res.*, **28**, 207

8. Atkins, H. J. B., Hayward, J. L., Klugman, D. J. and Wayte, A. B. (1972). Treatment of early breast cancer: a report after ten years of clinical trial. *Brit. Med. J.*, **2**, 423

9. Urban, J. A. (1971). Significance of internal mammary lymph node metastases in breast cancer. *Am. J. Roentgenol.*, **111**, 130

10. Cole, M. P. (1964). The place of radiotherapy in the management of early breast cancer: a report of two clinical trials. *Brit. J. Surg.*, **51**, 24

11. Nissen-Meyer, R. (1965). Castration as part of the primary treatment for operable female breast cancer. *Acta Radiol. (Diagn.). Suppl.*, **249**, 1

12. Ravdin, R. G., Lewison, E. F., Slack, N. H., Gardner, B., State, D. and Fisher, B. (1970). Results of a clinical trial concerning the worth of prophylactic oophorectomy for breast carcinoma. *Surg. Gynec. & Obst.*, **131**, 1055

13. Fisher, B., Ravdin, R. G., Ausman, R. K., Slack, N. H., Moore, G. E. and Noel, R. J. (1968). Surgical adjuvant chemotherapy in cancer of the breast: results of a decade of co-operative investigation. *Ann. Surg.*, **168**, 337

14. Hayward, J. L. and Bulbrook, R. D. (1965). The value of urinary steroid estimations in the prediction of response to adrenalectomy or hypophysectomy. *Cancer Res.*, **25**, 1129

15. Barlow, D. and Meggitt, B. F. (1968). Clinical indices to the response rate of advanced breast cancer to bilateral adrenalectomy and oophorectomy. *Brit. J. Surg.*, **55**, 809

16. Anglem, T. J. and Leber, R. E. (1971). Characteristics of ten year survivors after radical mastectomy for cancer of the breast. *Am. J. Surg.*, **121**, 363

17. Bulbrook, R. D. (1971). Some basic difficulties in attempting to predict response to therapy by endocrine assay. *Nat. Cancer Inst. Monogr.*, **34**, 39

18. MacMahon, B., Cole, P., Lin, M., Lowe, C. R., Mirra, A. P., Ravnihar, B., Salber, E. J., Valoras, V. G. and Yuasa, S. (1970). Age at first birth and breast cancer risk. *Bull. Wld. Hlth. Org.*, **43**, 209

19. Logan, W. P. D. (1953). Marriage and childbearing in relation to cancer of the breast and uterus. *Lancet*, **ii**, 1199

20. Report to the Council on Drugs (1960). Androgens and oestrogens in the treatment of disseminated mammary cancer. *J. Amer. Med. Ass.*, **172**, 1271

21. Hayward, J. L. (1957). An evaluation of some factors affecting oestrogen response in the treatment of advanced cancer of the breast. *Guy's Hospital Reports*, **106**, 254

22. Myers, M. H., Axtell, L. M. and Zelen, M. (1966). *Clinical Evaluation in Breast Cancer*, p. 215. (J. L. Hayward and R. D. Bulbrook, editors.) London and New York: Academic Press

23. Galasko, C. S. B. (1972). Skeletal metastases and mammary cancer. *Ann. Roy. Coll. Surg.*, **50**, 3

24. Shapiro, S. (1973). Evaluation of thermography in mass screening for breast cancer. *First Breast Cancer Task Force Working Conference*, Williamsburg, Virginia. U.S. Dept. of Health, Education and Welfare, Nat. Cancer Inst., U.S.A.

25. Kusama, S., Spratt, J. S., Donegan, W. I., Watson, F. R. and Cunningham, C. (1972). The gross rates of growth of human mammary carcinoma. *Cancer*, **30**, 592

26. Cady, B. (1972). Changing patterns of breast cancer. *Arch. Surg.*, **104**, 266

27. Bagshawe, K. D., Golding, P. R. and Orr, A. H. (1969). Choriocarcinoma after hydatidiform mole. Studies related to effectiveness of follow-up practice after hydatidiform mole.

28. Hayward, J. L. and Bulbrook, R. D. (1966). *Clinical Evaluation in Breast Cancer.* London and New York: Academic Press

29. Brennan, M. J. (1966). *Indices of Response to Breast Cancer Therapy*, p. 141. (J. L. Hayward and R. D. Bulbrook, editors.) London and New York: Academic Press

30. Atkins, H. J. B., Falconer, M. A., Hayward, J. L., MacLean, K. S., Schurr, P. H. and Armitage, P. (1960). Adrenalectomy and hypophysectomy for advanced cancer of the breast. *Lancet*, **i**, 1148

31. Atkins, H. J. B., Hayward, J. L., Klugman, D. J. and Wayte, A. B. (1972). Treatment of early breast cancer: a report after ten years of a clinical trial. *Brit. Med. J.*, **2**, 423

32. Bulbrook, R. D. and Greenwood, F. C. (1957). Persistence of urinary oestrogen excretion after oöphorectomy and adrenalectomy. *Brit. Med. J.*, **1**, 662

33. Young, Stretton (1957). Pituitary necrosis due to implants of radioactive gold and yttrium. *Lancet*, **i**, 548

34. Annotation (1970). Hormone profiles and discriminant function in cancer. *Lancet*, **ii**, 1070
35. Abe, O. (1971). Ablative hormone therapy in advanced breast cancer. *Clin. Orth. Surg.*, **6**, 614
36. Cutler, S. J. (1966). *Clinical Evaluation in Breast Cancer*, p. 215. (J. L. Hayward and R. D. Bulbrook, editors.) London and New York: Academic Press
37. Miller, H. and Durant, J. A. (1968). The value of urine steroid hormone assays in breast cancer. *Clin. Biochem.*, **1**, 287
38. Myers, M. H., Axtell, L. M. and Zelen, M. (1965). The use of prognostic factors in predicting survival for breast cancer patients. Joint Meeting of American Statistical Association, Biometric Society (ENAR) and Institute of Mathematical Statistics, Philadelphia, Pa. U.S.A.
39. Wolff, B. (1966). Histological grading in carcinoma of breast. *Brit. J. Cancer*, **20**, 36
40. Lundmark, C. (1972). Breast cancer and elastosis. *Cancer*, **30**, 1195
41. Shivas, A. A. and Douglas, J. G. (1972). The prognostic significance of elastosis in breast carcinoma. *J. Roy. Coll. Surg. Edin.*, **17**, 315
42. Gross, F., Mahringer, W., Trebbin, H. and Bohle, A. (1965). The significance of Barr Bodies in cancer of the breast. *Germ. Med. Mth.*, **10**, 12
43. Hienz, H. A. (1965). Die zell kernmorphilogische Geschlechtserkennung au tumoren. *Med. Welt.*, **50**, 2803
44. Perry, M. (1972). Evaluation of breast tumour sex chromatin (Barr Body) as an index of survival and response to pituitary ablation. *Brit. J. Surg.*, **59**, 731
45. Atkin, N. B. (1972). Modal deoxyribonucleic acid value and survival in carcinoma of the breast. *Brit. Med. J.*, **1**, 271
46. Strong, J. A., Brown, J. B., Bruce, J., Douglas, M., Klopper, A. I. and Loraine, J. A. (1956). Sex-hormone excretion after bilateral adrenalectomy and oophorectomy in patients with mammary carcinoma. *Lancet*, **ii**, 955
47. McAllister, R. A., Sim, A. W., Hobkirk, R., Stewart, H., Blair, D. W. and Forrest, A. P. M. (1960). Urinary oestrogen after endocrine ablation. *Lancet*, **i**, 1102
48. Hayward, J. L., Bulbrook, R. D. and Greenwood, F. C. (1961). Hormone assays and prognosis in breast cancer. *Memoirs of the Soc. of Endrocin.*, **10**, 144
49. Irvine, W. T., Aitken, E. H., Rendleman, D. F. and Folca, P. J. (1961). Urinary oestrogen measurements after oöphorectomy and adrenalectomy for advanced breast cancer. *Lancet*, **ii**, 791
50. Young, S., Bulbrook, R. D. and Greenwood, F. C. (1957). The correlation between urinary oestrogen and vaginal cytology. *Lancet*, **i**, 350
51. Dilman, V. M., Berstein, L. M., Bobrov, Y. F., Bohman, Y. U., Kovaleva, I. G. and Krylova, N. V. (1968). Hypothalamopituitary hypersensitivity and endometrial carcinoma. *Am. J. Obst. Gyn.*, **102**, 880
52. Leman, H., Wotiz, H. H., Parsons, L. and Mozden, P. J. (1966). Reduced oestriol excretion in patients with breast cancer after endocrine therapy. *J. Amer. Med. Ass.*, **196**, 1128
53. MacMahan, B., Cole, P., Brown, J. B., Aoki, K., Lin, T. M., Morgan, R. W. and Woo, N-C. (1971). Oestrogen profiles of Asian and North American women. *Lancet*, **ii**, 900
54. Wynder, E. L., Lucas, J. C. and Farrow, J. (1963). A comparison of survival rates

between American and Japanese patients with breast cancer. *Surg. Gyn. Obstet.*, **117**, 196

55. Shucksmith, H. S., Bonser, G. M., Dossett, J. A., Henderson, W. R. and Jull, J. W. (1960). A method of selection of patients with advanced breast cancer for hypophysectomy or adrenalectomy: a preliminary report. *Proc. Roy. Soc. Med.*, **53**, 901

56. Boot, L. M. (1970). Prolactin and mammary gland carcinogenesis; the problem of human prolactin. *Int. J. Cancer*, **5**, 167

57. Pearson, D. H., Llerena, O., Llerena, L., Molina, A. and Butler, T. (1969). Prolactin-dependent rat mammary cancer. A model for man? *Trans. Ass. Amer. Physicians*, **82**, 225

58. Wang, D. Y., Hallowes, R. C., Smith, R. H., Amor, V. and Lewis, D. J. (1972). A biochemical comparison of the lactogenic effects of prolactin and growth hormone on mouse mammary gland in organ culture. *J. Endocr.*, **52**, 349

59. Hadfield, G. (1957). The nature and origin of the mammotrophic agent present in normal female urine. *Lancet*, **i**, 1058

60. Baron, D. N., Gurling, K. J. and Smith, E. J. R. (1958). Effect of hypophysectomy in advanced carcinoma of the breast. *Brit. J. Surgery*, **45**, 593

61. Segaloff, A., Gordon, D., Carabasi, R. A., Horwitt, B. N., Schlosser, J. V. and Murison, P. J. (1954). Hormonal therapy in cancer of the breast. VII. Effect of conjugated estrogens (equine) on clinical course and hormonal excretion. *Cancer*, **7**, 758

62. McCalister, A. and Welbourn, R. B. (1962). Stimulation of mammary cancer by prolactin and clinical response to hypophysectomy. *Brit. Med. J.*, **1**, 1669

63. Sinha, Y. N., Selby, F. W., Lewis, U. J. and Vanderlaan, W. P. (1973). A homologous radioimmunoassay for human prolactin. *J. Clin. Endocr. Metab.*, **36**, 509

64. Boyns, A. R., Cole, E. N., Griffiths, K., Roberts, M. M., Buchan, R., Wilson, R. G. and Forrest, A. P. M. (1973). Plasma prolactin in breast cancer. *Europ. J. Cancer*, **9**, 99

65. Newsome, J. F., Timmons, R. L., Van Wyk, J. and Dugger, G. S. (1971). Pituitary stalk section for metastatic carcinoma of the breast. *Ann. Surgery*, **174**, 769

66. Pearson, I. H., Llerena, O., Samaan, N. and Gonzalez, D. (1968). *Prognostic Factors in Breast Cancer*, p. 421. (A. P. M. Forrest and P. B. Kunkler, editors.) Edinburgh and London: E. S. Livingstone

67. Greenwood, F. C., James, V. H. T., Meggit, B. F., Miller, J. D. and Taylor, P. H. (1968). *Prognostic Factors in Breast Cancer*, p. 409. (A. P. M. Forrest and P. B. Kunkler, editors.) Edinburgh and London: E. S. Livingstone

68. Beck, J. C., Blair, A. J., Griffiths, M. M., Rosenfeld, M. W. and McGarry, E. E. (1966). In search of hormonal factors as an aid in predicting the outcome of breast carcinoma. *Proc. Can. Cancer Res. Conf.*, **6**, 3

69. Schubert, K., Bacigalupo, G. and Frankenberg, G. (1961). Der corticosteroid-spiegel ales blutes bei nastopathie und brustkrebs unter ACTH balastung. *Arch. Geschwulstforsch.*, **17**, 108

70. Benard, H., Bourdin, J. S., Saracino, R. T. and Seeman, A. (1962). Etude des 17-hydroxycorticosteroides plasmatiques dans 52 cas de cancer du sein. *Annls. Endocr.*, **23**, 15

71. Jensen, V., Deshpande, N., Bulbrook, R. D. and Doouss, T. W. (1968). Adrenal function in breast cancer: production and metabolic clearance rate of cortisol in patients with early or advanced breast cancer and in normal women. *J. Endocr.*, **42**, 425

72. Doouss, T. W. and Deshpande, N. (1968). *In vivo* perfusion of the human adrenal gland and ovary in patients with mammary cancer. *Brit. J. Surg.*, **55**, 673

73. Deshpande, N., Jensen, V., Carson, P., Bulbrook, R. D. and Doouss, T. W. (1970). Adrenal function in breast cancer: biogenesis of androgens and cortisol by the human adrenal gland *in vivo*. *J. Endocr.*, **47**, 231

74. Deshpande, N., Jensen, V., Bulbrook, R. D. and Doouss, T. W. (1967). *In vivo* steroidogenesis by the human adrenal gland. *Steroids*, **9**, 393

75. Saez, S. (1971). Adrenal function in cancer: relation to the evolution. *Europ. J. Cancer*, **7**, 381

76. Bishop, M. C. and Ross, E. J. (1970). Adrenocortical activity in disseminated malignant disease in relation to prognosis. *Brit. J. Cancer*, **24**, 719

77. Ghosh, P. C., Lockwood, E. and Pennington, G. W. (1973). Abnormal excretion of corticosteroid sulphates in patients with breast cancer. *Brit. Med. J.*, **1**, 328

78. Dao, T. L. (1969). *The Human Adrenal Gland and its Relation to Breast Cancer*, p. 99. (K. Griffiths and E. H. D. Cameron, editors.) Cardiff: Alpha Omega Alpha

79. Chou, C-Y. and Wang, C. W. (1939). Excretion of male sex hormone in health and disease. *Chinese J. Physiol.*, **14**, 151

80. Allen, B., Hayward, J. L. and Merivale, W. H. H. (1957). The excretion of 17-ketosteroids in the urine of patients with generalized carcinomatosis secondary to carcinoma of the breast. *Lancet*, **i**, 496

81. Bulbrook, R. D., Greenwood, F. C. and Hayward, J. L. (1960). Selection of breast cancer patients for adrenalectomy or hypophysectomy by determination of urinary 17-hydroxycorticosteroids and aetiocholanolone. *Lancet*, **i**, 1154

82. Atkins, H., Bulbrook, R. D., Falconer, M. A., Hayward, J. L., MacLean, K. C. and Schurr, P. H. (1964). Urinary steroid estimations in the prediction of response to adrenalectomy or hypophysectomy. *Lancet*, **ii**, 1133

83. Atkins, H., Bulbrook, R. D., Falconer, M. A., Hayward, J. L., MacLean, K. C. and Schurr, P. H. (1968). Urinary steroids in the prediction of response to adrenalectomy or hypophysectomy: a second clinical trial. *Lancet*, **ii**, 1263

84. Armitage, P., McPherson, C. K. and Copas, J. C. (1969). Statistical studies of prognosis in advanced breast cancer. *J. Chron. Dis.*, **22**, 343

85. Sarfaty, G. and Tallis, M. (1970). Probability of a woman with advanced breast cancer responding to adrenalectomy and hypophysectomy. *Lancet*, **ii**, 685

86. Wilson, R. E., Crocker, D. W., Fairgrieve, J., Bartholomay, A. F., Emerson, K. and Moore, F. D. (1967). Adrenal structure and function in advanced carcinoma of the breast. *J. Am. Med. Ass.*, **199**, 474

87. Wilson, R. E. and Moore, F. D. (1968). *Prognostic Factors in Breast Cancer*, p. 399. (A. P. M. Forrest and P. B. Kunkler, editors.) Edinburgh and London: E. S. Livingstone

88. Wilson, R. E., Piro, A. J., Aliopoulios, M. A. and Moore, F. D. (1971). Treatment of metastatic breast cancer with a combination of adrenalectomy and 5-fluorouracil. *Cancer*, **28**, 962

89. Juret, P., Jayem, M. and Flaisler, A. (1961). A propos de 150 implantations

d'yttrium radio-actif intrahypophysaires dans le traitement du cancer du sein au stade avance. *J. Chir. (Paris)*, **87**, 409

90. Kumaoka, S., Sakauchi, N., Abe, O., Kusama, M. and Takatani, O. (1968). Urinary 17-ketosteroid excretion of women with advanced breast cancer. *J. Clin. Endocr.*, **28**, 667

91. Fotherby, K. A., Sellwood, R. A. and Burn, J. I. (1970). Urinary steroid excretion in patients with advanced breast cancer. *Brit. J. Surg.*, **57**, 859

92. Sarfaty, G., Tallis, M. and Pitt, P. (1973). Basic results of a study of bilateral adrenalectomy for advanced breast cancer. Urinary steroids and related data in 148 patients. *Aust. Med. J.* (in Press)

93. Hobkirk, R. and Forrest, A. P. M. (1957). Urinary steroid patterns in breast cancer. *Lancet*, **i**, 636

94. Sim, A. W., Hobkirk, R., Stewart, H. J., Blair, D. W. and Forrest, A. P. M. (1960). Urinary 17-ketosteroids and their fractions in women with breast cancer treated by endocrine surgery. *Brit. J. Cancer*, **14**, 460

95. Ahlquist, K. A., Jackson, A. W. and Stewart, J. C. (1968). Urinary steroid values as a guide to progress in breast cancer. *Brit. Med. J.*, **1**, 217

96. Bulbrook, R. D., Hayward, J. L. and Thomas, B. S. (1964). The relation between the urinary 17-hydroxycorticosteroids and 11-deoxy-17-oxosteroids and the fate of patients after mastectomy. *Lancet*, **i**, 945

97. Hayward, J. L. and Bulbrook, R. D. (1968). Urinary steroids and prognosis in breast cancer. *Prognostic Factors in Breast Cancer*, p. 383. (A. P. M. Forrest and P. B. Kunkler, editors.) Edinburgh and London: E. S. Livingstone

98. Bulbrook, R. D. (1972). Hormones and Breast Cancer Workshop. Breast Cancer Task Force, Nat. Cancer Inst., Bethesda, Maryland, U.S.A.

99. Wade, A. P., Davis, J. C., Tweedie, M. C. K., Clarke, C. A. and Haggart, B. (1969). The discriminant function in early carcinoma of the breast. *Lancet*, **i**, 853

100. Cameron, E. H. D., Griffiths, K., Gleave, E. N., Stewart, H. J., Forrest, A. P. M. and Campbell, H. (1970). Benign and malignant breast disease in South Wales. A study of urinary steroids. *Brit. Med. J.*, **4**, 768

101. Jensen, E. V. and Jacobson, H. I. (1962). Basic guides to the mechanism of oestrogen action. *Recent. Progr. Horm. Res.*, **18**, 387

102. Folca, P. J., Glascock, R. F. and Irvine, W. T. (1961). Studies with tritium-labelled hesoestrol in advanced breast cancer. *Lancet*, **ii**, 796

103. King, R. J. B., Smith, J. A. and Steggles, A. W. (1970). Oestrogen-binding and the hormone responsiveness of tumours. *Steroidologia*, **1**, 73

104. Terenius, L. (1972). Parallelism between oestrogen binding capacity and hormone responsiveness of mammary tumours in GR/A mice. *Europ. J. Cancer*, **8**, 55

105. James, F., James, V. H. T., Carter, A. E. and Irvine, W. T. (1971). A comparison of *in vivo* and *in vitro* uptake of oestradiol by human breast tumours and the relationship to steroid excretion. *Cancer Res.*, **31**, 1268

106. Feherty, P., Farrer-Brown, G. and Kellie, A. E. (1971). Oestradiol receptors in carcinoma and benign disease of the breast: an *in vitro* assay. *Brit. J. Cancer*, **25**, 697

107. Bulbrook, R. D. (1966). Measurement of hormonal status. *Clinical Evaluation in Breast Cancer*, p. 77. (J. L. Hayward and R. D. Bulbrook, editors.) London and New York: Academic Press

108. Braunsberg, H., James, V. H. T., Irvine, W. T., James, F., Jamieson, C. W., Sellwood, R. A., Carter, A. E. and Hulbert, M. (1973). Prognostic significance of oestrogen uptake by human breast cancer tissue. *Lancet*, **i**, 163

109. Englesman, E., Persijn, J. P., Korsten, C. B. and Cleton, F. J. (1973). Oestrogen receptor in human breast cancer tissue and response to endocrine therapy. *Brit. Med. J.*, **2**, 750

110. Jensen, E. V. (1972). *Hormones and Breast Cancer Workshop*. Breast Cancer Task Force, Nat. Cancer Inst., Bethesda, Maryland, U.S.A.

111. Jensen, E. V., Block, G. E., Smith, S., Kyser, K. and De Sombre, E. R. (1971). Oestrogen receptors and breast cancer response to adrenalectomy. *Prediction of Response in Cancer Therapy*, T. C. Hall, editor. *N.C.I. Monograph*, **34**, 55

112. Wittliff, J. L., Hilf, R., Brooks, W. F., Savlov, E., Hall, T. and Orlando, R. (1971). Specific oestrogen-binding capacity of the cytoplasmic receptor in normal and neoplastic tissue of humans. *Cancer Res.*, **32**, 1973

113. Mioduszewska, O., Koszarowski, T. and Gorski, C. (1968). The influence of hormones on breast cancer *in vitro* in relation to the clinical course of the disease. *Prognostic Factors in Breast Cancer*, p. 347. (A. P. M. Forrest and P. B. Kunkler, editors.) Edinburgh and London: E. S. Livingstone

114. Salih, H., Flax, H. and Hobbs, J. R. (1972). *In vitro* oestrogen sensitivity of breast cancer tissue as a possible screening method for hormonal treatment. *Lancet*, **i**, 1198

115. Stoll, B. A. (1972). *In vitro* oestrogen sensitivity of breast cancer. *Lancet*, **i**, 1339

116. Flax, H., Salih, H., Newton, K. A. and Hobbs, J. R. (1973). Are some women's breast cancers androgen dependent? *Lancet*, **i**, 1204

117. Heuson, J. C. and Tagnon, H. J. (1973). Androgen dependence of breast cancers. *Lancet*, **ii**, 203

118. Rose, D. P. (1967a). Tryptophan metabolism in carcinoma of the breast. *Lancet*, **i**, 239

119. Rose, D. P. (1967b). The influence of sex, age and breast cancer on tryptophan metabolism. *Clin. Chim. Acta*, **18**, 221

120. Davis, H. L., Leklem, J. E., Carlson, I. and Brown, R. R. (1970). Correlation of urinary steroids and tryptophan and kynurenine metabolism in patients with breast cancer. *Proc. Amer. Ass. Cancer Res.*, **11**, 19

121. Bell, E. D., Mainwaring, W. I. P., Bulbrook, R. D., Tong, D. and Hayward, J. L. (1971). Relationships between excretion of steroid hormones and tryptophan metabolites in patients with breast cancer. *Am. J. Clin. Nutr.*, **24**, 694

122. Bell, E. D., Tong, D., Mainwaring, W. I. P., Hayward, J. L. and Bulbrook, R. D. (1972). Tryptophan metabolism and recurrence rates after mastectomy in patients with breast cancer. *Clin. Chem. Acta*, **42**, 445

123. Davis, H. L. and Brown, R. R. (1969). Tryptophan metabolism and hormonal response in breast cancer patients. *Proc. Amer. Ass. Cancer Res.*, **10**, 10

124. Davis, H. L., Brown, R. R., Leklem, J. and Carlson, I. H. (1973). Tryptophan metabolism in breast cancer. Correlation with urinary steroid excretion. *Cancer*, **31**, 1061

125. Rose, D. P. and Randall, Z. C. (1972). Tryptophan metabolism in early and advanced breast cancer and carcinoma of the cervix. *Clin. Chem. Acta*, **40**, 276

126. Hilf, R. (1971). Will the best model of breast cancer please come forward? *Nat. Cancer Inst. Monograph*, **34**, 43

127. Smith, J. A., King, R. J. B., Meggitt, B. F. and Allen, L. N. (1970). Enzyme activity, acidic nuclear proteins and prognosis in human breast cancer. *Brit. Med. J.*, **2**, 698

128. Dao, T. and Libby, P. R. (1969). Conjugation of steroid hormones by breast cancer tissue and selection of patients for adrenalectomy. *Surgery*, **66**, 162

129. Dao, L. and Libby, P. R. (1971). Enzymic synthesis of steroid sulphate by mammary cancer and its clinical implications. *Nat. Cancer Inst. Monograph*, **34**, 205

130. Doll, R. and Kinlen, L. (1970). Immunosurveillance and cancer: epidemiological evidence. *Brit. Med. J.*, **4**, 420

131. Kaplan, H. S. (1971). Role of immunological disturbance in human oncogenesis: some facts and fancies. *Brit. J. Cancer*, **25**, 620

132. Mackay, W. D. and Baum, M. (1968). The role of immune factors in breast cancer. *Prognostic Factors in Breast Cancer*, p. 319. (A. P. M. Forrest and P. B. Kunkler, editors.) Edinburgh and London: E. S. Livingstone

133. Hughes, L. E. and Mackay, W. D. (1965). Suppression of the tuberculin response in malignant disease. *Brit. Med. J.*, **2**, 1346

134. Williams, W. J. and Roberts, M. M. (1968). Delayed hypersensitivity in breast cancer. *Prognostic Factors in Breast Cancer*, p. 331. (A. P. M. Forrest and P. B. Kunkler, editors.) Edinburgh and London: E. & S. Livingstone

135. Mitchell, R. J. (1972). The delayed hypersensitivity response in primary breast carcinoma as an index of host resistance. *Brit. J. Surg.*, **59**, 505

136. Jacobs, D., Houri, M., Landon, J. and Merrett, T. G. (1972). Circulating levels of immunoglobulin E in patients with cancer. *Lancet*, **ii**, 1059

137. Augustin, R. and Chandradasa, K. D. (1973). Circulating levels of IgE in patients with cancer. *Lancet*, **i**, 102

138. Laurence, D. J. R. and Neville, M. A. (1972). Foetal antigens and their role in the diagnosis and clinical management of human neoplasma: a review. *Brit. J. Cancer*, **26**, 335

139. Stonehill, E. H. and Bendich, A. (1970). Retrogenetic expression: the reappearance of embryonal antigens in cancer cells. *Nature*, **228**, 370

140. Lo Gerfo, P. (1972). Tumour-associated antigen levels in patients with colon and breast carcinoma. *Rev. of Surgery*, **29**, 224

141. MacSween, J. M., Warner, N. L., Bankhurst, A. D. and Mackay, I. R. (1972). Carcinoembryonic antigen in whole serum. *Brit. J. Cancer*, **26**, 356

142. Chan, S. P., Maca, R. D., Levine, P. H. and Ting, R. C. (1971). Immunologic studies of human breast cancer. 1. Serum reactivity against a lymphoid cell line (Belev) derived from a breast cancer patient as detected by complement-fixation test. *J. Nat. Cancer Inst.*, **47**, 511

143. Whittaker, M. G. and Clark, C. G. (1971). Depressed lymphocyte function in carcinoma of the breast. *Brit. J. Surg.*, **58**, 717

144. Krant, M. J., Brandrup, C. S., Greene, R. S., Pochi, P. E. and Strauss, J. S. (1968). Sebaceous gland activity in breast cancer. *Nature*, **217**, 463

145. Burton, J. L., Cunliffe, W. J. and Shuster, S. (1970). Increased sebum excretion in patients with breast cancer. *Brit. Med. J.*, **1**, 665

146. Wang, D. Y., Bulbrook, R. D., Guillebaud, J. and Lewis, A. (1972). *Europ. J. Cancer*, **8**, 381

147. Lee, Y-T. (1971). The ABO blood groups and results of therapeutic oophorectomy for advanced carcinoma of the breast. *Surgery Gynec. Obstet.*, **123**, 871

148. Anderson, D. E. (1971). Some characteristics of familial breast cancer. *Cancer*, **28**, 1500

149. Morosini, P., Lee, E-G., Jones, M. ·N., Vessey, M. P., Heinonen, O. P., Nevanlinna, H. R. and Svinhufvud, U. L. M. (1972). Breast cancer and the S blood-group system. *Lancet*, **i**, 411

150. Haenszel, W. (1964). Contributions of end results data to cancer epidemiology. *Nat. Cancer Inst. Monograph*, **15**, 21

151. Mackay, E. N. and Sellers, A. H. (1965). Breast cancer at the Ontario clinics 1938–1956. A statistical review. Medical Statistical Branch, Ontario Dept. of Health, 1965

152. MacMahon, B., List, N. D. and Eisenberg, H. (1968). Relationship of survival of breast cancer patients to parity and menopausal status. *Prognostic Factors in Breast Cancer*, p. 56. (A. P. M. Forrest and P. B. Kunkler, editors.) Edinburgh and London: E. & S. Livingstone

153. Morrison, A. S., Lowe, C. R., MacMahon, B., Warram, J. H. and Yuasa, S. (1972). Survival of breast cancer patients related to incidence risk factors. *Int. J. Cancer*, **9**, 470

154. Annotation (1972). Benign and malignant breasts. *Lancet*, **ii**, 218

155. Silverberg, S. G., Chitale, A. R. and Levitt, S. H. (1972). Prognostic implications of fibrocystic dysplasia in breasts removed for mammary carcinoma. *Cancer*, **29**, 574

156. Brennan, M. J., Bulbrook, R. D., Deshpande, N., Wang, D. Y. and Hayward, J. L. (1973). Urinary and plasma androgens in benign breast disease. Possible relation to breast cancer. *Lancet*, **i**, 1076

157. Izuo, M., Okagaki, T., Richard, R. M. and Lattes, R. (1971). *Cancer*, **28**, 620

158. Bulbrook, R. D., Hayward, J. L. and Spicer, C. C. (1971). Relation between urinary androgens and corticoid excretion and subsequent breast cancer. *Lancet*, **ii**, 395

Index

217